Trauma Reco

CW00493477

Strategic Guide to Reducing Stress, and Inner Body Fears to Overcome Trauma

By

William Winder

The Star Publications

Table of Contents

About the Author

William Winder is a parenting expert. He has almost 15 years of experience in his field. He gives realistic solutions supported by in-depth, evidence-based research and advocates for a strict yet supportive positive parenting approach. He is a renowned author, family counselor, and specialist who helps families by disseminating his ideas on bringing up cooperative and resilient children. He offers a fresh and optimistic view of your existing family dynamic with doable strategies that give you strength and faith.

He assists you whether you are searching for a quick suggestion to get you through a meltdown or want to go deeper to improve your family life. His delivery is quick, cordial, and motivating. Today's busy parents will find his deep insights easy to understand and immediately useful.

Preface

According to a recent study, 61% of teenagers (aging between 13 to 17 years) have experienced at least one traumatic incident in their lives. 19% have been through three or more traumatic events.

These statistics shouldn't come as much of a surprise when you think about how difficult life can be for teens. Adolescence is a period of change and development. Teens are also being exposed to a broader range of experiences during the sensitive teen years. This exposure occurs naturally as they progress toward maturity and grow over time.

Ask a teenager about their life, and they will tell you about their daily struggles. The same would be the case for a parent of a teenager. Now imagine the struggles of an adolescent child and his parents who have been through some kind of trauma or are going through one! The struggle gets tenfold in this case.

Given the importance of the teenage years for growth and development, it is imperative to deal with any trauma that has been burdening the life of a teen and his family.

This book is for all those teens who feel the extra pressure from any traumatic incident in their life and wish to fix it. Or you could probably be the parent of a traumatized teen reading this book. You can utilize the knowledge given in this book to help your kid to recover.

Introduction

Jason, a 15-year-old kid, came to my clinic with a history of bullying. He attended a high school in a small community, where the majority of the kids came from families who belonged to the upper-middle class and resided in suburban regions. Because of the tight-knit nature of the local communities, the vast majority of kids, parents, and instructors were familiar with one another by name.

Jason was upset that his classmates were making fun of him and calling him names while interacting with him on various social media platforms. In addition, Jason experienced physical bullying, which consisted of three lads punching him in the stomach and threatening to do it again if he informed anybody about it. The incident was witnessed (in person) by one of the instructors, and when she questioned the boy about it, Jason revealed to her that he had also been bullied through social media platforms. After that, the homeroom instructors had a discussion with the three older kids who were bullying Jason; all of them were 18 years old. They denied that they had done anything improper or harmful; they didn't perceive it as being harmful at all. They saw it as simply being harmless jokes. They vowed that, that would be the last time they did it. This had been traumatic for Jason, and he had to seek therapy.

The story of Jason is rather a common occurrence that many teens go through in their lives. I get to hear parents who struggle with their teens when their children refuse to open up and communicate about what has been troubling them. It is indeed not easy for young kids to talk about their pain regarding certain traumatic events with their parents. In some cases of trauma, such as a natural disaster or the sudden death of a loved one in the family, it is easier for parents to point out and observe the change in their child's behavior. But with hidden cases of trauma such as sexual abuse or bullying, the parents may be clueless about what has been bothering their child. In any case, professional counseling can help a great deal.

Although the subject of trauma or PTSD is not new to be addressed but dealing with teen trauma has unfortunately not been addressed much in the past. I believe with the rapidly changing dynamics of our social and technological evolution, the subject of teen trauma needs to be highlighted and talked about more than ever. I have decided to write this book with a goal in mind to help teens to recover from the effects of their traumatic experiences.

Reading this book, you'll learn about the fundamentals of trauma, how traumatic experiences rewire the brain, and what other effects trauma may have. The later part of the book will help you to learn about some practical ways to deal with trauma and recover from it. You'll also find some activities and exercises used in psychotherapy to deal with trauma.

No matter if you're a teen reading this book to get some help or a parent to help your teen, this book will provide you with all the essential knowledge to curb issues caused by trauma. So let's get started! Recover from trauma and start living a fearless and fulfilling life.

Chapter 1: Learning the Basics of Trauma

Henry is a youngster who is 13 years old and lives in the same house as his mother and elder brother, who is 16 years old. Henry's mother was the target of an attempted murder committed by his father. Two years earlier, Henry watched his father stabbing his mom in the stomach in front of him. In the years leading up to this incident, Henry and his brother were eyewitnesses to a number of episodes of domestic violence that were committed by their father. Their father was subsequently arrested for this incident.

The present state of henry's mother is miserable. She has a long history of significant depression. She is currently having an episode and spends much of her day in bed. Henry's brother has been arrested a number of times for various violent crimes and thefts of automobiles. Additionally, his brother has brutally attacked their mother on two separate occasions. Henry's mother is afraid of being harmed if she attempts to place limits on her elder son's conduct.

The relationship between Henry and his brother is strained. Fist fights have broken out on a regular basis at home as a result of the many disagreements that take place there. After being knocked unconscious by his brother, Henry lives in constant terror that his brother may have another episode of "losing it." The poor boy has regular flashbacks of all times when his father used to hit his mother. As a result, he has an excessive startle response, is always on guard, and is paranoid about being harmed. He has trouble falling asleep, which results in frequent nightmares, and he also has a hard time concentrating while he is awake. As a result of poor concentration, he did not pass the sixth grade since he struggled to pay attention in class. This is the second year in a row that he is at risk of failing the sixth grade, and he has informed his therapist that he plans to take his own life if he is unsuccessful at school.

Henry's case is an extreme one in nature since it involves the elements of crime such as theft attempts by his brother and murder attempt by his father. But many teens may be traumatized by some event that is otherwise considered normal. Consider the death of a grandparent that lives in the same house as the teen. If a teen child is attached to the grandparent, the death may cause extreme psychological disturbance to the child. This may lead to building symptoms of trauma. Whereas, for many children, such an incident may have a temporary effect and may not result in significant trauma.

In some cases, the traumatic experiences may lead to the development of post-traumatic stress disorder or PTSD. But there are also some other disorders that have symptoms similar to PTSD, but they are not PTSD precisely. So what are the criteria to qualify for proper trauma diagnosis? What are the types of trauma? What is PTSD and other stressor-related disorders? And what does trauma look like in teens? These are the questions that I am going to answer in this chapter.

1.1 Defining Trauma

Trauma is a response to a very upsetting or disturbing event that overpowers a person's ability to cope, leads to feelings of helplessness, erodes one's sense of self, and restricts one's ability to feel the full range of emotions and experiences.

It affects people of all backgrounds equally, and it is widespread around the globe. According to the findings of a study on world mental health performed by the World Health Organization (WHO) in 26 distinct countries, at least one-third of the more than 125,000 individuals questioned had been through some kind of traumatic event.

There is no objective definition that can be used to determine which experiences may result in post-traumatic symptoms; nonetheless, the themes generally entail a loss of control, abuse of authority, helplessness, suffering, disorientation, and pain. It is not necessary for the incident to reach the level of war, natural catastrophe, or personal attack for it to deeply influence a person and for their experiences to change. The traumatic experiences that might trigger post-traumatic symptoms in a person can vary greatly from one individual to another. In point of fact, it is quite subjective, and it is essential to keep in mind that it is characterized more by its reaction than by its cause.

1.2 Types and Symptoms of Trauma

A person who is exposed to traumatic events may react in a variety of ways. It's possible that they are in a state of shock, profound sorrow, or denial about the situation. In addition to the quick or short-term response, trauma may also give birth to a number of longer-term responses, such as emotional dysregulation, nightmares, impulsiveness, flashbacks, and impact on relationships. These longer-term reactions can occur years after the initial traumatic event. In addition to the psychological symptoms, those who have been through traumatic experiences may also have physical symptoms, such as fatigue, headaches, and nausea. It's possible that some people will be far more impacted than others. People who are greatly affected by a traumatic experience may have a tough time moving on with the rest of their life because they are stuck in the emotional effect that the trauma has on them. The expression of trauma over a prolonged period of time may sometimes result in a psychological condition known as post-traumatic stress disorder (PTSD).

Although there is a wide variety of experiences that may be classified as traumatic; nevertheless, there are several typical situations that are commonly deemed traumatic. The following are some examples of the kinds of traumatic experiences that a person could have at some time in their life:

• Abuse
• Car accident
• Assault
• Loss of a family member or friend
• Divorce
• Abandonment by family members or by parents.
• Imprisonment
• Natural catastrophes
• Job loss
• Injury to the body
• Rape
• Violence
• Illness of a grave nature
• Terrorism
• Being a witness to a homicide, an accident, or a death

Acute trauma, chronic trauma, and complex trauma are the three primary types of traumas.

Acute Trauma

It is often the outcome of a single traumatic experience, such as being in an accident, being raped, being assaulted, or experiencing a natural catastrophe. The occurrence is severe enough to put the person's emotional as well as bodily safety in jeopardy. The experience leaves a mark on the person's psyche that will not easily be forgotten. It has the potential to influence both the way a person thinks and acts if it is not treated with professional assistance. In most cases, symptoms of acute trauma manifest themselves as:

- Excessive worry or a state of panic
- Irritation
- Confusion
- Incapacity to have a pleasant night's sleep or insomnia in extreme cases
- A feeling of estrangement from one's immediate environment
- A lack of trust that is irrational and unreasonable
- An inability to concentrate on one's job or academic pursuits
- Neglect of personal hygiene and appearance
- Aggressive behavior

Chronic Trauma

It occurs when a person is subjected to a series of traumatic experiences that are stressful and last for a lengthy amount of time or are repeated over a prolonged period of time. Chronic trauma may be the consequence of a major disease that lasts for a long period of time, sexual abuse, domestic abuse, bullying, or exposure to harsh conditions such as a war.

Chronic trauma may develop from a number of different episodes of acute trauma as well as from acute trauma that is not addressed. The symptoms of chronic trauma often manifest after a significant amount of time has passed, sometimes even years after the traumatic incident. The symptoms are very upsetting, and they might emerge as emotional outbursts that are erratic or unexpected, anxiety, excessive rage, flashbacks, weariness, bodily pains, headaches, and nausea. It's possible that these people have difficulty with trusting others, which is why they don't have solid relationships or employment. It is essential for the individual to get assistance from a licensed psychologist in order to recover from the upsetting symptoms.

Complex Trauma

It is the outcome of being exposed to a wide variety of stressful experiences or incidents on repeated occasions. In most cases, the occurrences take place within the framework of a personal connection (one that exists between individuals). It might make a person feel like they're stuck. Complex trauma may often have a profound effect on a person's mental state. People who have been the targets of childhood abuse, neglect, marital violence, family disagreements, and other recurrent events, such as civil unrest, are at a higher risk of developing this condition. It has an impact on the individual's general health, as well as on their relationships and their performance in the workplace or school.

No matter what kind of traumatic experience a person has been through, if they are having trouble recovering from the upsetting events, they need to get professional psychological assistance as soon as possible. The individual who has been through a traumatic experience may lead a more fulfilled life with the assistance of a trained therapist.

1.3 Trauma, PTSD, and Other Stressors-Related Disorders

Throughout the course of our lives, each and every one of us experience stress. A person is said to have experienced trauma when their capacity to deal with the aftermath of a highly stressful or upsetting incident is compromised as a result of an intense emotional reaction to the event.

It is important for those who have witnessed or experienced trauma, as well as their loved ones, to be aware of the signs and symptoms of post-traumatic stress disorder (PTSD), as well as the ways in which it can be treated, and how to seek help, even though trauma does not always directly lead to post-traumatic stress disorder (PTSD).

There is a spectrum of intensity and effects associated with the trauma; in fact, roughly one in three individuals who have been exposed to severe trauma also suffer from post-traumatic stress disorder (PTSD).

Despite the fact that post-traumatic stress disorder is most often associated with troops returning from war zones having experienced the atrocities of war, this disorder may affect anybody who has observed or experienced horrific, life-threatening, or life-changing experiences. According to the National Center for PTSD, post-traumatic stress disorder (PTSD) is a prevalent condition that affects 10% of women and 4% of men at some time in their life.

People of any age may develop post-traumatic stress disorder (PTSD). There is no one who is immune to the effects that trauma has on the human brain. PTSD might mean something different to each individual, yet it still has the same devastating effects on their lives.

It is possible for an individual to have a unique experience of post-traumatic stress due to the unique nature of the traumatic event that they went through; even the symptoms of post-traumatic stress may differ from person to person. In some instances, the manifestation of symptoms might be quite rapid. In the case of certain individuals, the onset of symptoms and subsequent diagnosis may take decades. There is a delayed start of symptoms for many people, which occurs either when the brain is no longer as distracted or when the individual has the time to comprehend what has occurred.

There is no conclusive explanation as to why some persons who suffer traumatic events acquire post-traumatic stress disorder (PTSD) while others do not. One's vulnerability to developing post-traumatic stress disorder (PTSD) may be increased by a combination of factors, some of which include the following:

•   A history of traumatic events, which may include aspects such as the frequency with which traumatic events occurred and the intensity of those traumatic events.
•   Anxiety and depression tendencies that run in the family
•   Reaction based on feelings and emotions (temperament)

- The manner in which your brain controls the hormones and substances that are secreted by your body as a reaction to stressful experiences
- Some vocations, such as being a soldier, nurse, doctor, law enforcement officer, or fireman, subject workers to greater trauma than other jobs do.

The experience of a traumatic or stressful incident that results in psychological suffering is the defining characteristic of trauma and stressor-related conditions.

In the past, trauma or stressor-related conditions were simply labeled as yet another kind of anxiety disorder. The discovery that these conditions were not founded on anxious or fear-based symptoms, on the other hand, brought a shift in this perception. People who were traumatized or who suffered from stress-related conditions predominantly displayed symptoms such as anhedonia (the inability to experience pleasure), dysphoria (a feeling of uneasiness or discontent), dissociative symptoms, and externalization of rage along with violent symptoms. Individuals who suffer from trauma or stressor-related disorders may still exhibit anxiety or fear-based symptoms, but they are not the core symptoms of the condition.

Because of this, the Diagnostic and Statistical Manual of Mental Disorders, Fifth Edition (DSM-5), has given disorders associated with traumatic experiences and other stressors its own chapter. Although post-traumatic stress disorder (PTSD) is perhaps one of the most well-known trauma and stressor-related disorders, there are a number of additional conditions that also fall into this category, including the following:

Acute Stress Disorder

A person may develop acute stress disorder if they are confronted with a perceived or real danger to their life, major injury, or sexual assault, regardless of whether or not they were personally involved in the incident or simply witnessed it. There are five categories that describe different sorts of symptoms, and these categories include intrusion, negative mood, avoidance, dissociation, and arousal. The symptoms of acute stress disorder are quite similar to those of post-traumatic stress disorder (PTSD); however, acute stress disorder manifests itself during the first month after exposure to the traumatic event. It is possible to forestall the development of PTSD by promptly treating ASD.

Adjustment Disorders

Behavioral or emotional symptoms in reaction to a circumstance that happened within three months of the onset of the symptoms are what distinguish adjustment disorders from other mental health conditions. These symptoms are often defined as being out of proportion for the degree of the stressor and as being the source of severe social, occupational, or other sorts of impairment to one's day-to-day life. Individual symptoms may vary and may include but are not limited to depressive episodes, anxious episodes, a combination of depressive and anxious episodes, and behavioral issues.

Disinhibited Social Engagement Disorder (DSED)

Disinhibited social engagement disorder (DSED) is a condition that affects children and is defined by the children behaving in a very familiar manner with people they don't know. Children who have DSED do not have a fear of approaching and engaging with persons they do not know, do not check back with their guardian after wandering away, and are prepared to leave without hesitation when asked to do so by an unknown person. A child may acquire DSED if they are socially neglected, if they have frequent changes in their main caregivers, or if they are brought up in an environment that hinders their capacity to build selective attachments.

Reactive Attachment Disorder (RAD)

Kids between the ages of 9 months and five years might be diagnosed with reactive attachment disorder, which is defined by emotionally detached behavior towards adult caregivers. Children who have RAD seldom look for or react to attempts to console them when they are upset; they have a little emotional and social response to others; and they may be irritated, unhappy, or scared during non-threatening encounters with caregivers. A pattern of inadequate care, such as the one which occurs in situations of child abuse or with children in the foster care system who fail to create secure attachments, may lead to the development of reactive attachment disorder (RAD).

Unspecified Trauma and Stressors Related Disorder

When there is not enough information to determine a precise diagnosis, a diagnosis of unidentified trauma and stressor-related condition may be made instead. It is possible to use it to characterize symptoms that are related to trauma disorders that produce discomfort and impairment but that do not match all of the criteria necessary for diagnosis.

1.4 Trauma in Teens

Children go through a great deal of emotional development while they are in their teenage years. From infancy through adolescence, there is a dramatic shift in both their perspectives of the reality around them and their position within it. Teens are susceptible to a variety of problems if they are exposed to traumatic events when their minds and emotions are still in a formative stage. Teenagers who have experienced traumatic events may lash out, carry out activities that are harmful, and begin using substances such as alcohol or drugs as a means of numbing their pain. It is essential for the loved ones of adolescents to provide support for them and seek out options that might assist them in coping with traumatic experiences in positive ways.

A person may experience trauma as a consequence of either being a victim of violence or watching another person being a victim of violence. It's a sad reality that up to 5 million children and teenagers in the United States alone go through something traumatic every single year. A staggering one-fourth of all children who are ever born will, by the time they reach the age of 18, have been a victim of sexual assault. The vast majority of incidents are not brought to light; it is estimated that 86 percent of sexual assaults and 65 percent of physical assaults committed against teenagers go unreported.

Deep agony, humiliation, and guilt are the aftereffects of traumatic experiences. Even if many traumatic incidents aren't documented, victims and their closed loved ones nonetheless feel the effects of it. It's possible that adolescents who experience a dramatic shift in their mental state or conduct have been traumatized. It is tough for adults to ask for assistance, and it may be much more difficult for teenagers to do so.

Adolescents who have been through traumatic events but have not received therapy for those experiences are much more prone to participate in risky behavior and activities. Girls who have been through traumatic experiences are more prone to get pregnant at a young age and to participate in sexually unsafe conduct. It is not uncommon for traumatized adolescents to engage in risky behaviors such as running away from home, skipping school, or abusing substances. PTSD is the most common mental health condition that may be brought on by exposure to traumatic events. The symptoms of post-traumatic stress disorder (PTSD) affect an estimated twenty million youngsters.

Adults have a tough time dealing with traumatic situations and digesting the terrible feelings that are triggered by these kinds of events. Teenagers, on the other hand, do not yet have the emotional responses or the cognitive ability necessary to properly process trauma in the absence of outside help. While many adolescents who have been through traumatic experiences may act out and display problematic behaviors, others will have a distinct set of symptoms. Problems falling asleep, withdrawing from friends and family, and having trouble focusing in class are all quite typical. These problems may have a significant influence on a teen's ability to make plans for their future when they graduate from high school.

In addition, it is normal for traumatized adolescents to have severe emotional outbursts that seem to be inappropriate for the setting. Some people internalize their suffering, which may lead to depression and the addiction of substances like alcohol or narcotics. These difficulties may potentially land traumatized teenagers in legal jeopardy, aggravating their troubles. When teenagers are left to their own devices to deal with the effects of traumatic experiences, it may result in emotional scars that last a lifetime, but it can also have other ramifications in the actual world.

1.5 Trauma, Adolescence, and the Brain Development

The brain is a magnificent organ, and it continues to grow and develop until the early to mid-twenties. Children and adolescents who go through traumatic experiences are more likely to have problems with their brain development, especially with the abilities associated with executive functioning. Teens who have been through traumatic experiences may have difficulties developing the following skills:

- The capacity for time management and organization of schedules
- Impulse control
- Prioritizing tasks
- Make decisions, and then act in accordance with those decisions.
- Remembering and recalling the details
- Exhibit and acknowledge the appropriate emotional reactions or behavioral responses

A teen is more likely to suffer a wide variety of unpleasant thoughts and feelings if they have been through traumatic experiences and have not received enough help. Memories that are upsetting and persistent might make it difficult for a person to think clearly and feel at peace with themselves. Trauma and the pain it creates may lead to high levels of stress if they are not managed properly. Stress is a major factor in the development of addiction and may be a precipitating factor as well. In the short term, abusing substances like alcohol or drugs may help minimize unpleasant thoughts and sensations. However, in the long run, substance misuse exacerbates the effects of traumatic events. It is possible to safeguard teenage victims of trauma against the aforementioned dangers and repercussions by providing them with the necessary assistance as soon as possible.

Every aspect of human behavior is controlled by the brain, from involuntary actions like inhaling oxygen to more conscious actions like engaging in a conversation or giggling at jokes. Therefore, in order to understand how to develop relationships with teenagers, it is necessary to have an awareness of how the brain may change over the course of a lifetime as a result of aging and previous experiences, as well as how these changes in the brain influence behavior.

For example, throughout adolescence, the brain goes through substantial changes that have an effect on how an adolescent perceives themselves in relation to the environment surrounding them. As adolescents make the journey from childhood to adulthood, they go through a number of important life changes, including more independence, more personal relationships, difficult and crucial choices, and other major life-altering experiences. The following are some of the ways a teen's brain is attempting to get ready for this:

- **It is "use it or lose it" for your cells:** In order for it to be ready for maturity, the brain of a teenager goes through a period of massively increased cell production. This provides the brain with the chance to learn new abilities. On the other hand, if these extra brain cells are not properly stimulated and/or if they are not guided in a forgiving and loving manner by an adult, they will ultimately die off. Despite the fact that this does not exclude the development of talents in coming times, it may significantly slow down the process.
- **The maturation of the prefrontal cortex:** A significant amount of growth takes place in the prefrontal cortex region of the brain during adolescence. This is the region of the brain that is responsible for self-control, decision-making, organization, prioritization, restricting inappropriate behaviors, activating appropriate behaviors, empathizing with others, and many other related traits. However, while the prefrontal cortex is still growing, the amygdala, which is a more emotional region of the brain, takes control. This means that the majority of circumstances and dialogues are perceived and processed largely via the emotional mind instead of the logical mind.
- **Reconstruction of the neural pathways:** Different regions of the brain need to be in conversation with one another in order for us to be able to think, perform, or feel more than one thing simultaneously. Myelin, a

layer that helps speed up communication along the neural pathway between different sections of the brain, increases throughout the adolescent years. Because of this transition, serotonin production (which is a hormone that improves mood) slows down, which means that teens are more likely to feel irritation and have relatively low moods.

These changes, along with a great number of others, are caused by a child's biology and take place independently of their environment. However, traumatic experiences, abuse, abandonment, major life changes, and other environmental factors or experiences in the past make a contribution to how the brain develops during this critical period. This is because of the reason that the brain relies on familiar behaviors or areas of the brain that are frequently used to determine which parts of the brain to reinforce and which parts of the brain to weaken during this period of mental growth.

To rephrase it in other words, kids learn to figure out and build their own techniques to fulfill the wants which are not being satisfied, and with the passage of time, those tactics alter the brain. Consider the following example: when a kid is undernourished, their brain is preoccupied with finding the next meal and figuring out how to prepare it. As time passes, the kid learns whatever actions are required to get that meal, and the areas of the brain that are responsible for those behaviors and actions get stronger. This is an evolutionary method of guaranteeing that the kid will live and be fed despite any obstacles that may arise.

In a similar manner, when a child is subjected to repeated traumatic experiences, his brain develops certain behaviors that help it to survive the high levels of stress and remain constantly alert. Over time, these behaviors change the brain in the following ways: the parts of the brain that control anxiety and fear grow in order to protect the child, while other parts of the brain that control and regulate more critical or logical thinking shrink. It's possible that these two regions of the brain are at odds with each other, which may lead to flashbacks as well as difficulties understanding or recognizing emotional reactions. At some point, the neural circuits linked with fear become so persistently stimulated that the brain produces permanent memories, alterations in attitude, and adjustments in perception as a result of the constant activation. This implies that even after a kid has established safety, the coping strategies he once used to endure traumatic experiences continue to exist. This may result in responses to particular triggers that are unexpected or out of control, problems processing or comprehending the consequences of actions, and other potentially troublesome behaviors such as hoarding, screaming, or angry outbursts. Thus, the problematic behaviors are the results of a child's brain making its best effort to meet the child's requirements in the face of a lack of reliable assistance.

In the brains of people who have been through traumatic experiences, specific noises, scents, sights, tastes, body gestures, facial expressions, activities, seasons, and phrases are associated with the traumatic events in order to better prepare the brain for any possible future threats. After some time has passed and it has been determined that the environment is safe, the brain will continue to register some cues as harmful, which may cause an emotional reaction.

When seen from the outside, a teenager who has been triggered by something may seem to be "acting out." This is because their response appears to be exaggerated and out of their control, and it may be difficult to determine what triggered it.

In case of any action or behavior that is the result of a traumatic experience, parents and other caregivers need to take advantage of this situation to remind teenagers that they have support from them no matter how they act or whatever the reasons behind those behaviors. After the adolescent has regained their composure and sense of security, you should work with them to figure out what caused them to react the way they did and how you both can approach similar situations in the future in a more productive manner by using language that is developmentally appropriate. Get in the car, go on a stroll, or play a video game together, and while you're doing one of those things, start a conversation by saying something like, "I saw that something occurred this morning that made you feel awful. We may make an effort to determine what it is about. Can you recall what happened in the moments just before you became angry with me?"

Loss of biological family members, neighborhoods, homes, pet animals, and friends may all have a significant impact on a child's brain development, as can early neglect or abuse, unsuccessful reunification or numerous changes in foster care, trauma, or the absence of a safe attachment figure (someone whom the child could securely get attached with). As a consequence of this, the manner in which a kid behaves in social situations, emotionally and intellectually, may not be in line with the child's chronological age or physical age. They may form patterns of relationships that are either unstable or intense, while at the same time, they oppose being interdependent or connected with other individuals in their community. They may also experience problems with their cognition and memory, which may have a negative impact on how well they do at home, in school, and on the job. Because of this, it's possible for teens to be mature and well-developed in certain areas yet be behind their age level in other domains.

In a nutshell, a child's capacity to work through their ideas, feelings, and behaviors is altered and, in some manner, slowed down by the time they reach puberty. Regardless of whether or not a kid has been exposed to traumatic experiences, the child's brain will undergo chemical and structural changes that may result in behaviors that may appear strange or problematic. However, kids who have been through traumatic situations must adapt to these typically occurring alterations in addition to dealing with the consequences that the experiences have had on their development.

Trauma and teen years combine to disrupt a child's relationships and personal sense of self, and the foundation of successful intervention and therapy is re-establishing and restoring the connection.

1.6 Childhood Adversities, ACEs, and Trauma

Childhood adversity is a broad phrase that refers to a wide variety of conditions or events that constitute a substantial danger to the physiological or psychological wellbeing of a kid. Child abuse and neglect, bullying, major accidents or injuries, prejudice, extreme poverty, and communal violence are all examples of common forms of adversity that children may face throughout their formative years. According to research, such events may have substantial repercussions, particularly when they take place at a young age, are persistent and/or severe, or compound over the course of one's lifetime. For instance, the consequences of early trauma may become physiologically ingrained throughout critical phases of development, which can eventually lead to permanent difficulties with both physical and mental health. However, children who experience adversity are not automatically doomed to have negative results, and the majority of children are able to recover when they receive the appropriate support, most notably the regular presence of a kind caregiver who is warm and sympathetic.

Adverse childhood experiences (ACEs) are a subset of childhood adversity. The term "adverse childhood experiences" or ACEs was developed by researchers Robert Anda, Vincent Felitti, and their colleagues in their foundational study that was performed from 1995 to 1997. The researchers polled adults about their experiences with seven different types of adversities during their formative years. These included emotional, sexual, and physical abuse; seeing a mother experiencing domestic violence; living with somebody who was mentally ill, living with someone who abused drugs or alcohol, and having a member of the household incarcerated. According to the findings of the research, the more adverse childhood experiences (ACEs) adults reported from their youth, the worse their mental and physical health outcomes were (e.g., substance misuse, heart diseases, depression). Since that initial study, the word ACEs has come to be used to refer to a variety of different lists of adverse experiences. The current Adverse Childhood Experiences (ACEs) study, which is funded by the Centers for Disease Control and Prevention, takes into account instances of physical and emotional neglect, as well as parental separation or divorce. Other studies have also taken into account instances of social disadvantage such as poor economic conditions, being homeless, discrimination, community violence, and historical trauma.

No ACEs list or screening tool can detect all childhood adversities, yet, those lists that do not consider adversity connected to socioeconomic inequality are likely to ignore children who belong to certain racial or ethnic groups that are adversely affected. It is of equal importance to evaluate the state of each child's wellbeing in order to determine the kind(s) of services that would be of the greatest use to that particular child. A kid who has gone through adverse childhood experiences (ACEs) but is able to function normally should not be over-treated; hence it is important to get a complete picture of the child.

One of the outcomes that may result from being subjected to adversity is trauma. When a person sees an incident or set of circumstances as being particularly terrifying, hurtful, or dangerous — either mentally, physically, or both — they have experienced trauma. This may happen when the person is exposed to the event or conditions. Soon after a traumatic event, a child may begin to experience intensely negative feelings, such as fear or helplessness, as well as physiological symptoms, such as a rapid heartbeat, wetting the bed, or stomach aches. These feelings and symptoms may persist for a significant amount of time after the initial exposure. Certain forms of adversity experienced throughout childhood are more prone to trigger traumatic responses in children. These include the unexpected death of a family member, the occurrence of a natural catastrophe, the experience of a major auto accident, or the occurrence of a school shooting. Other traumatic events that may occur throughout childhood include parental separation or divorce, which tends to be connected with a greater degree of heterogeneity in children's responses and may or may not be seen as traumatic by the kid. Experiencing traumatic events as a child is linked to issues across a variety of aspects of development. However, every kid reacts uniquely to traumatic experiences because of the unique combination of individual, familial, and environmental risks and protective variables that make up that child. For instance, two children who go through the same kind of difficulty may react in different ways: One person could bounce back quickly without experiencing major difficulty, while another might develop posttraumatic stress disorder (PTSD) and need the assistance of a trained professional.

A child may suffer toxic stress if they are subjected to adversity that is intense, long-lasting, and severe (for example, chronic neglect, domestic abuse, severe economic difficulty), yet they do not get appropriate assistance from an adult who is responsible for their care. In particular, adversities that occur throughout childhood, such as ACEs, have the potential to over-activate the child's stress response system, which, over time, may wear down both the body and the brain. This over-activation is known as toxic stress, and it is the major way in which a child's development and wellbeing are negatively impacted when they are subjected to adversity. The degree to which a child's stress response to adversity gets toxic and leads to major physical and mental health issues in adulthood also relies on the child's biological make-up (for example, genetic vulnerabilities, previous experiences that have harmed the stress response system, or inhibited healthy expression of genes), as well as the specifics of the adverse events or situations (e.g., duration, intensity, or when a caregiver was the abuser, etc.).

The growing recognition that childhood adversity, especially ACEs, may induce trauma and toxic stress and affect children's mental and physical health gives a chance to take proper action. For instance, caregivers and other professionals in child and family service systems may educate themselves on trauma-informed care and put it into practice in these settings. Nevertheless, we must also be careful to avoid focusing just on adverse childhood experiences (ACEs) since doing so might prevent us from comprehending the entire scope of adverse childhood experiences and establishing the other reasons for trauma in teens.

Chapter 2: Effects of Trauma on Teens

Although the degree to which an individual is affected by trauma is subjective, nevertheless, trauma may have severe effects on some individuals. Because it is so distressing to be reminded of the traumatic event or events, a person who has survived a traumatic incident may find themselves going to considerable measures to avoid any reminders of the experience. For instance, you may not want to think about or speak about the traumatic experience. You might also choose to avoid particular persons or locations that bring up memories of what happened. When it comes to some individuals, the avoidance is so ingrained that they are unable to recall significant portions of the experience. You may also feel as if you are not connecting with other people, which may lead to a loss of interest in life. A significant number of people who have PTSD report feeling emotionally numb, in particular when it comes to their positive emotions. You may also believe that there is no use in making plans for the future or that there is a possibility that you will not live to enjoy pleasant things in your life. These effects may prove to be worse for teens. Take the case example of Nancy.

Nancy is a student, and she is nineteen years old. At the age of eighteen, she became the victim of sexual assault committed by the coach of the basketball team she played for. In the days leading up to the assault, he paid Nancy a considerable lot of attention, often praising her and offering to drive her back to her dormitory. Nancy appreciated his attention, but she saw the interaction as nothing more than innocent flirting. Following the incident, Nancy made the decision to leave the basketball team immediately. She hasn't been seen in regular attendance at school for more than six months, and she hasn't answered calls from her previous teammates who have tried to get in touch with her.

She is seldom seen out with her pals and has given up on dating. She used to take pleasure in watching sports on TV, but now she avoids doing so because it makes her weep excessively and prompts her to reflect on the mistreatment she received from her coach. She has expressed her feelings of betrayal, anger, and loneliness and says she has serious reservations about her ability to trust anybody, especially a male, ever again.

Children whose families and surroundings do not provide them regular security, protection, and comfort may develop strategies of coping that enable them to live and function in their day-to-day life. These children are at a higher risk of developing mental health issues later in life. For example, they may have an abnormally high sensitivity to the feelings and behaviors of other people, and they may constantly be observing the actions and emotions of the adults in their environment in order to predict how those adults would act. It's possible that they hide their own feelings from others, never letting anybody know when they're worried, upset, or frustrated. When there is a constant risk of bodily or mental harm, it makes sense for a person to adapt in ways like these via learning. These adjustments are no longer beneficial to the kid when he or she becomes an adult and comes into contact with environments and relationships that are secure; in fact, they may be unproductive and interfere with the child's ability to live, love, and be loved. There are many different ways in which teenage victims of trauma might be affected. The after-effects of trauma may linger on and affect the teen in its adult life. In this chapter, I am going to throw light on some of these effects.

2.1 Attachment and Relationships

After going through a traumatic experience, many individuals discover that their connections with the people around them are altered. It is not uncommon for the overwhelming conditions brought on by traumatic occurrences to have an effect on a person's relationships with their friends, family, workplace, and other people. Even while these responses are specific to each individual and are based on the particular traumatic event that they have had, the majority of individuals have certain responses that are common to what has occurred to them. A person's feeling of security and safety in the world is severely tested whenever a traumatic incident takes place. It's possible that their faith in the future will be challenged, that their perspective on the purpose of life will shift, and that both the way they think about themselves and the way they feel about themselves will alter. These emotions may be mirrored in a number of ways within a person's relationships.

The experience of having lived through traumatic experiences may leave a person with the anticipation of experiencing danger, betrayal, or possible injury within new or existing relationships. It may be difficult for survivors to trust people, even those individuals whom they have previously placed their confidence in, since they may feel confused and vulnerable about what is safe. Fear of getting hurt in an unsafe environment may make it difficult to become close to others.

People may also experience anger as a result of feeling powerless and losing control over aspects of their life, which may lead them to become violent or attempt to exert control over others. A person who has been through traumatic experiences may feel threatened more quickly, which may lead to increased levels of anger and aggressive behavior. When confronted with danger, it is only normal for a person to respond with aggressive defensive behavior. It is also possible for an individual's concept of who he or she is to be altered as a result of the experience. Trauma survivors may feel great shame, feel unlovable or awful in some manner, or guilty about what happened to them. A person may have the impression that no one can completely comprehend what has taken place, or they may be concerned that it will be too taxing to share their experiences with those who are particularly close to them. Some people develop a habit of isolating themselves from other people, pulling away from their friends, family, and life in general, and experiencing feelings of distance, separation, or detachment as a result. Others may have feelings of anxiety or fear with respect to other people, see those other people as having power or influence over them, or find it easy to feel abandoned or rejected.

A significant number of people who have survived traumatic experiences report feeling emotionally numb and report having difficulty experiencing or expressing good feelings within the context of a relationship. Additionally, physical closeness may be more challenging, and some survivors of traumatic events may discover that it is difficult, if not impossible, to establish a sexual relationship that is satisfying to them. The normal emotions might be perplexing or scary for a trauma survivor.

When a child or a teen is subjected to traumatic events at a young age, for example, when they are sexually molested by a trusted family member, the most fundamental components of safety and trust within a primary relationship are weakened. The person's capacity to feel peaceful and to anticipate caring, responsive, and comfortable relationships in adult life is negatively impacted as a result of the disruptions in the earliest attachments. There is a possibility that memories and sentiments of betrayal, grief, guilt, secrecy, humiliation, and threats to one's physical integrity may emerge or become a part of subsequent relationships. Some individuals, especially those who have been neglected or abused as children, may fail to form fundamental trust and secure bonds in their relationships. This may be because of the trauma they have experienced as a kid.

It is impossible to exaggerate the value of a child's tight bond with a caregiver. Children develop a sense of the world as either safe or unsafe, as well as an understanding of their own value as individuals through the development of attachment relationships with significant figures in their lives. These relationships teach children how to trust and have faith in others, how to control their emotions, and how to interact with people in the world. Children learn that they cannot depend on the assistance of others when they have interactions with other people that are unpredictable or unstable. When a kid's main caretakers exploit and abuse them, the youngster grows up believing that they are awful people and that the world is a terrible place.

The majority of neglected or mistreated children struggle to form a strong, healthy bond with a caregiver. Stress is more likely to affect children who don't have strong bonds with their caregivers. They have difficulty managing and expressing their emotions, and their responses to circumstances are sometimes aggressive or otherwise inappropriate. Our capacity to have healthy, supportive connections with friends and loved ones is contingent on our ability to form such ties in our own families. A teen who has had several traumatic events throughout his life may struggle to maintain healthy romantic connections, healthy friendships, and healthy interactions with those in positions of authority, such as teachers and law enforcement personnel.

2.2 Emotional Responses

Some people who have experienced traumatic events have trouble regulating and controlling their emotions, including anger, anxiety, grief, and shame. This is especially true when the traumatic event occurs at a young age. However, in people who are older and functioning well before the trauma, this kind of emotional dysregulation is often short-lived and is an acute response to the trauma rather than a continuing pattern. In other words, it is not a pattern that persists over time. Self-medication, more specifically the misuse of substances, is one of the techniques that traumatically affected individuals employ in an effort to restore emotional control, despite the fact that, in the long run, it creates even more emotional dysregulation. Other methods of controlling one's emotions include repressing or denying feelings, engaging in risky or self-destructive activities, having an eating problem, engaging in obsessive behaviors such as gambling or overworking oneself, and so on. It is important to note that not all actions related to self-regulation are seen as having a negative connotation. In point of fact, some people find inventive, healthy, and productive ways to manage the intense feelings that are generated by traumatic experiences. This may include making a strong commitment to physical activity or founding an organization whose mission is to support survivors of a specific type of traumatic event.

When someone is exposed to traumatic stress, they may experience one of the two emotional extremes: experiencing either an abundance of emotion (overwhelmed) or an absence of emotion (numbness). Kids who have been through several traumatic experiences often struggle to recognize, communicate, and control their feelings, and they may have limited words for describing how they are feeling. They typically internalize and/or externalize their emotions in response to stress, and as a consequence, they may feel substantial levels of depression, anxiety, or rage. Their emotional reactions are likely to be erratic or explosive. A teen could shake, become angry, feel sad, or try to avoid anything that reminds him of the traumatic incident he experienced. It's possible that a teenager who has been through several traumatic experiences would find that reminders of those experiences are everywhere in his surroundings. When angry, such a youngster can have trouble calming down, frequent outbursts of strong emotion, and intense reactions. Since the traumatic experiences are often of a social or interpersonal nature, even contact with people who are just somewhat uncomfortable may function as memories of the traumatic event and set off significant emotional reactions. Such kids are typically guarded and alert in their dealings with others. They are also more prone to see circumstances as dangerous or stressful, having learned that this world is a horrible place where even close loved ones can't be trusted to protect you. This defensive position is helpful in protecting a person when that individual is under assault, but it may become troublesome in circumstances that do not necessitate such a severe reaction. Alternately, many youngsters learn to tune out to the dangers that are present in their surroundings, which leaves them susceptible to being victimized again.

Emotional regulation issues are quite common, and they may arise even in the absence of close personal connections. A good many of these youngsters have never been taught how to settle their own emotions after they have been agitated; therefore, they find it difficult to cope when faced with challenging situations. For instance, when faced with difficult assignments at school, they may feel so discouraged that they give up on even the smallest of the tasks. Children who are exposed to strong traumatic experiences at a young age have a higher risk of developing an irrational fear of many different things, including being afraid all the time. They also have a greater risk of suffering from clinical depression.

2.3 Physical Health – Brain and Body

When children reach the age of 18, they do not miraculously "get over" whatever traumatic experiences they have had. Recent research conducted by Harvard University found that traumatic events, toxic stress, and bad childhood experiences may permanently damage a child's body and brain, which can have major effects that last a person's whole life.

There are several ways in which a child's growing system might get overwhelmed by the effects of trauma. The fluctuation in hormone levels is the first aspect to consider. The "stress hormones" adrenaline and cortisol assist you in responding to a perceived danger or threat by directing blood circulation to key muscle groups and by-passing the portion of the brain that is responsible for thinking in order to activate the part of the brain that is responsible for survival.

These hormones keep your blood sugar levels raised, which may lead to type 2 diabetes. They also disturb your immune function and inflammatory response system that can contribute to developing lupus, multiple sclerosis, abdominal obesity, osteoarthritis, depression, and limit your capacity to fight off infections.

Alterations in hormone levels that occur in childhood, a time in life when brain growth is at its most rapid pace, have the potential to have a profound effect not just on the structure and function of the brain but also on other organs, leading to lifelong issues with both physical and mental health.

The second way that traumatic experiences may influence your body and brain is by causing alterations to your immune system. The immune system provides defense against infections, allergic reactions, and inflammatory responses by acting on different organs, tissues, and cell types.

Trauma is associated with thymus involution, shrinkage of lymph node and spleen, raised stress hormone levels, and telomere shortening, all of which decrease immunity and promote inflammation.

Inflammation and impaired immunity raise the risk of cancer, diabetes, cardiovascular disease, depression, anxiety, viral infections, autoimmune disorders, asthma, and allergies.

Alterations in one's nervous system may also be brought on by traumatic experiences. At birth, each of us has around 100 billion neurons, also known as brain nerve cells; this number represents the vast majority of the neurons we will ever possess. The formation of synaptic connections between neurons is responsible for the development of vision, hearing, speech, and higher cognitive functions.

The continuous activation of stress hormones at a young age might impair neural pathways in the thinking center of the brain, which is devoted to learning and reasoning, hence restricting cognitive abilities.

Continuous trauma may reduce existing neural connections to the thinking section of the brain while strengthening neural pathways to the survival section, bypassing the thinking half and leaving some youngsters less capable of dealing with hardship as they grow older.

Trauma also has the potential to alter your epigenetics. The field of research known as epigenetics examines how factors such as a person's environment and experiences may modify which genes are active and which are dormant. It is possible, for instance, that you were born with the potential to be tall and self-assured; yet, if you are malnourished as a kid and subjected to abuse, it is probable that you will develop into an adult who is short and timid instead.

The epigenetic makeup of genes involved in mental health, drug addiction, obesity, immunological function, metabolic illness, and cardiovascular disease may be altered as a result of traumatic experiences.

The body's biological systems continue to develop from childhood into adulthood. The environment has a role in determining the normal operation of biological systems. It's possible that a child's immune system and the body's stress response systems won't develop correctly if they grow up in an environment where they are constantly or intensely stressed. Later on, when the kid or adult is subjected to even typical amounts of stress, these systems may behave instinctively as though the person is under acute stress. This may occur in both children and adults. When confronted with stressful circumstances, a person may, for instance, exhibit strong physiological reactions such as fast breathing or heart racing, or they may "shut down" altogether. These behaviors, although adaptive when confronted with a major danger, are out of proportion in the context of routine stress, and others often interpret them as "overreacting" or as unresponsive or distant from the situation.

The presence of stress in a setting may interfere with the normal development of the central nervous system. In neglectful situations, a lack of mental stimulation may prevent the brain from reaching its full potential. Children who have experienced several traumatic events throughout their lives may have a history of developing chronic or recurring bodily issues, such as headaches or stomach pain. It has been shown that adults who have experienced traumatic events as children are more likely to suffer from chronic bodily ailments and issues. They could participate in dangerous activities, which would make these problems much worse.

Youth who have been exposed to several traumatic experiences usually suffer from body dysregulation, which means they either overreact or underreact to sensory inputs. They might be hypersensitive to noises, scents, touch, or light, or they could be suffering from analgesia and anesthesia, in which case they are oblivious to pain, touch, or internal bodily sensations. As a consequence of this, individuals may harm themselves without experiencing any pain, suffer from physical issues without being aware that they have them, or, on the other hand, they may claim to have chronic discomfort in numerous body parts for which there is no physical explanation that can be identified.

2.4 Dissociation

Dissociation is a possible response that some individuals exhibit when confronted with traumatic or severely stressful events. Robin, for instance, has planned to skydive for the first time and is really anxious about it. Robin's hands are shaking, his pulse rate is extremely elevated, and his thoughts are all mixed up. While the aircraft is taking off, Robin experiences chest tightness and the sensation that the world is spinning slightly. In the last moments, before he leaps, he has the impression that what is taking place is not real, and his limbs seem shaky and distant. As he takes the plunge and starts to descend, Robin is unable to focus on what is going on around him because he is dazed and confused. Signs of dissociation include changed perceptions of both the body and the outer environment. Dissociating during skydiving is not uncommon since it might be one of the ways we defend ourselves against imagined threats. Peritraumatic dissociation is the term for Robin's case of dissociating amid an overpowering incident.

It is possible for someone to experience dissociation as a reaction to traumatic experiences or as a reaction to continuous exposure to stress. For instance, a trauma that happens as a result of the interactions between individuals in their relationships. Memory, a person's sense of identity, the manner in which the world is experienced, and the link to the physical body may all be impacted by dissociation. These impacts are able to be felt not just during but also after exposure to traumatic events. Dissociation is a coping technique that the body develops in order to control and protect itself from excessive emotions and suffering. This is a normal response that some people have to terrible circumstances, and it may be useful as a means to cope with the situation at the moment. But when it occurs often, intensively, or in circumstances where it is not helpful, dissociation may become a problem, distressing a young person and having a detrimental effect on his life. This may have a variety of effects on a person, including making it difficult for them to focus at school or work, having trouble acquiring new information or remembering it, and giving them the impression that they are detached from their personal interactions with other people.

Children are more likely than adults to report having experienced dissociative phenomena. Early in one's childhood, it is possible to acquire it unknowingly as a method of defending oneself through times of suffering, physical and/or emotional abuse, terrifying events, and/or neglect. This is most prone to occur in children who have been subjected to lengthy or repeated traumatic experiences, as well as those who have been overwhelmed by events. A youngster who has been exposed to trauma for an extended period of time may develop the coping strategy of dissociation as a means of dealing with the effects of the trauma, and they may continue to use this method as they become older. When a kid experiences dissociation often throughout childhood, it may have a negative effect on the child's capacity to manage his emotions and stress as well as his sense of who he is. For young individuals, this may have detrimental effects in the future. Even as they get older, children may continue to disassociate anytime they are presented with a situation that causes them to feel uncomfortable feelings.

When the dissociative experience occurs in the absence of a traumatic experience, it is often possible for a person to be unaware that the dissociation they are going through is related to traumatic events from their past. It is essential to have this understanding since dissociation does not necessarily have to take place in conjunction with traumatic experiences. Dissociation triggers may not seem dangerous to others, but in young people who have experienced trauma firsthand, they may produce unpleasant emotions and/or memories for a variety of reasons. As the individual instinctively strives to protect oneself, these unpleasant sensations and/or memories might cause dissociation. When a young person and their loved ones have an understanding of the personal triggers that cause dissociation, it is much easier to comprehend the reasons why the young person dissociates and learn how to better handle triggers in the future. It's crucial to understand that with the correct help, recovering from dissociation and avoiding further episodes are both possible.

So what are the many forms of dissociation that young people are prone to experience? It is essential to comprehend that no two individuals will ever experience dissociation in precisely the same manner. This is due to the fact that the word "dissociation" denotes a diverse range of experiences. Each person's experience with problematic dissociation will be unique in terms of the severity, duration, and complexity of their symptoms. Problematic dissociation in adolescence might sometimes defy a predetermined diagnosis. Yet, it's crucial to understand that a young person's wellness and capacity for participation in everyday life might still be affected by these events. Young individuals may go through one of the phenomena given below, or more often, a mix of them.

Derealization: It is the state of feeling as if the world around you is an illusion. This state is referred to as the experience of derealization. People have reported having the sensation that the people and the world around them look two-dimensional, false, and/or lifeless. People may have a sense of disconnection from reality as if they are witnessing events unfold around them from a distant place or as if the events are happening in a movie.

Depersonalization: It is characterized by an altered feeling of one's own body, thoughts, actions, and/or sense of self. People have described feeling emotionally numb, floating, detached from bodily feelings, and/or acting as observers of their own bodies. It's also possible for people to have a strange perception of their own bodies, such as seeing their hands grow larger and smaller or having the sensation that their legs are shaky and far away.

Affected Memory: Dissociation may make it difficult for young people to pay attention to what is going on around them. Because of this, it is possible that they will be unable to recall part or all of the events that took place over that period of time. A young child may experience this and find it difficult to remember specifics of what happened within a certain time period.

Identity Alteration: A young person who experiences this kind of dissociation may experience a loss of identity. In addition to feeling significantly different from other aspects of themselves, young people may also realize that they are acting or thinking considerably different than they have been doing in the past. This changed sense of identity may or may not be recognized by individuals.

Somatization: Our body and dissociation have a complicated relationship with each other. Sometimes young individuals may endure bodily symptoms that cannot be explained by any recognizable ailment with their bodies. Some examples of these complaints include troubles with the stomach or other chronic aches. There may be a connection between these medical symptoms and psychological trauma.

2.5 Self-Regulation and Behavior

A youngster who has been through several traumatic experiences in the past may readily be triggered or "set off," and his reactions are more likely to be highly intense. The youngster could have trouble in self-regulating, which means he doesn't know how to calm down and might not be able to control his impulses or think through the repercussions of his actions before acting. As a consequence of this, children who have experienced any kind of trauma may exhibit behaviors that give the impression of being erratic, oppositional, explosive, or excessive. A youngster who was raised in fear of an abusive authority figure may respond defensively and angrily in reaction to the perceived blame or assault, or alternatively, he may at times be over-controlled, inflexible, and abnormally cooperative with adults. The fact that a youngster dissociates often will also have an effect on his conduct. It's possible that such a youngster would seem "spacey," aloof, or out of touch with the world around him. Children who have experienced several traumatic events are at a greater risk of engaging in high-risk behaviors, including but not limited to self-injury, hazardous sexual practices, and extreme risk-taking, such as driving a car at high speeds. They may also participate in unlawful activities like attacking others, theft, running away, gambling, or prostitution which raises the likelihood that they will be prosecuted by the juvenile justice system.

When it comes to assisting youngsters in developing the ability to moderate their physiological arousal, secure relationships with caregivers play an extremely important role. Perhaps the most severe consequence of neglect and trauma is the loss of the capacity to control the strength of emotions and impulses. It has been shown that the majority of children who are mistreated or neglected have dysfunctional attachment patterns. When a person is unable to control their feelings, it may lead to a variety of actions, most of which can be interpreted as efforts at self-regulation. These might include aggressive conduct against other people, harmful behavior toward oneself, eating disorders, and drug misuse. Self-definition and one's perspective on their environment are both influenced by their ability to control their internal states.

The inability of abused children to put their thoughts into words impedes their ability to respond in a flexible manner and encourages them to act out. Often, children who have been abused do not have the ability to discriminate between particular and general sentiments. In most cases, these behaviors occur simultaneously, which makes identification and therapy even more challenging. Affective dysregulation is something that can be helped by having safe attachments, having secure meaning systems, and having pharmaceutical treatments that increase the predictability of bodily reactions to stress. The capacity to describe terrible events symbolically encourages the regulation of fear and desomatization of painful memories.

2.6 Self-Concept and Future Orientation

Your connection with yourself, as well as the way you think about yourself and the issues you face, are both challenged and changed by traumatic experiences. Children acquire a sense of their own value from the responses of others, especially those who are closest to them. The feelings of self-worth and value that kids develop are strongly influenced by the people who care for them. Youngster who is neglected or abused will develop a hopeless and worthless sense of themselves. When a youngster is mistreated, they will often place the blame on themselves. It may seem more comfortable to blame oneself than it would be to acknowledge that the parent is untrustworthy and harmful. Children who have experienced several traumatic events often struggle with feelings of shame, remorse, low self-esteem, and a negative picture of themselves.

Prior to a traumatic life event, it's typical to have confidence in your capacity to make wise choices, manage your surroundings, and maintain your safety. These beliefs are dispelled by trauma and are replaced by other ones, such as the inability to trust your judgment. If you originally believed a circumstance, an individual, or behavior to be safe, but it turned out to be traumatic, it is simple to think that you are powerless to alter the situation, cannot control your destiny, and that forces outside of your control determine your safety.

These new beliefs may seem more true and compelling than the ones you had before the traumatic event, and as a result, they may lead to a diminished sense of control and safety. A natural consequence of this is an increase in the frequency and intensity of emotions of vulnerability and dread.

Increasing one's feeling of responsibility and control is a frequent strategy that may be used in an effort to regulate or lessen the heightened sensation of vulnerability and dread that one experiences. You can start blaming yourself for the terrible incident, despite the reality that no one who suffers a traumatic event causes it. You might also attempt to exert control over every aspect of your life, such as planning out every second of the day, trying to micromanage the lives of the people around you, or setting standards of perfection that are impossible to achieve.

Although it is completely normal that you would want to feel more in control of your life, these attempts frequently backfire and make you strive to control more aspects of your life. Not only will implementing a control agenda fail to provide the protection and security you want, but doing so will also demand a high psychological cost from you. Such excessive activities drain a person's body, mind, and soul, and exaggerated hopes breed harsh judgment and even self-hatred.

The harm that trauma does to your self-esteem also contributes to the bitterness and self-hatred that always develops after a traumatic life experience. It is a frequent misconception to feel that the traumatic event might have been avoided if the victim had been more intelligent, quicker, more physically capable, more vocal or just a better person overall. These erroneous assumptions, although reasonable, harm you by leading you to draw the mistaken conclusion that because the trauma occurred, you must have earned or caused it, and if you did, then all of the guilt and loathing you feel is justified.

These thoughts undermine your self-worth and fuel unkind perceptions of yourself to the extent that the resulting self-loathing may become intolerable and paralyzing, making you want to run away, vanish, constantly apologize for existing, or urgently try to show that you are deserving.

A youngster needs to feel confident in himself in order to look forward to the future with optimism and purpose. It takes optimism, self-assurance, and the capacity to perceive the purpose and worth in one's own activities to make plans for the future. Children who are subjected to violence in their families and communities have the understanding at a young age that they cannot trust others, that the world is not a safe place, and that they have no control over their surroundings. Their sense of competence is diminished by their beliefs about themselves, other people, and the world. Their pessimistic outlook prevents them from coming up with creative solutions to problems and prevents them from seizing chances to effect good change in their own life. A youngster who has had several traumatic experiences may believe that he is "damaged," helpless and that planning and taking meaningful action in the world is pointless. They have a hard time maintaining an optimistic outlook. As a result of having acquired the skills necessary to function in "survival mode," the kid lives from one moment to the next without stopping to reflect on, prepare for, or even fantasize about the future.

2.7 Long-Term Health Implications

There is a correlation between exposure to traumatic events in childhood and an increased risk of developing certain medical issues later in life. The Adverse Childhood Experiences (ACEs) Study (previously introduced in the first chapter) investigated the long-term effects of traumatic events that occurred during childhood and followed participants into adulthood. There were more than 17,000 participants in the ACE Study, whose ages ranged from 19 to 90. The researchers collected the patients' medical histories during the course of their study, in addition to data about the individuals' early experiences with abuse, violence, and compromised caregivers. According to the findings, roughly 66 percent of individuals with medical issues had at least one traumatic encounter, and of those, 69% had two or more traumatic experiences throughout their youth. The findings revealed a link between childhood trauma exposure, chronic diseases including cancer and heart disease, high-risk behaviors (such as unprotected sexual activity and smoking), and early death.

2.8 Cognitive Thinking and Learning

Children with profound trauma experiences may struggle to think coherently, reason, or solve problems. They may not be able to foresee the future, make predictions, or take appropriate action. All of a child's internal resources are directed toward surviving when they are raised in a constantly fearful environment. They may struggle to reason through a situation calmly and weigh all of the options when their bodies and thoughts have developed a chronic stress response state. It could be challenging for them to pick up new knowledge or skills. They could have trouble maintaining focus and attention, or they might get sidetracked by responses to traumatic recollections. They may have deficiencies in their capacity for abstract thought and language development. Many kids who have undergone repeated trauma have learning issues that could call for assistance in the classroom.

The experience of trauma may have a negative effect on a child's ability to learn, behave, and function socially, emotionally, and psychologically. Children struggle to reach their full potential when their basic physical needs, such as the need for protection, are not addressed. It is more likely that children will be unable to concentrate in class if they are preoccupied with their basic needs, such as the desire for a feeling of security, their emotional needs, and their physiological needs. These kids often struggle with behavioral issues, worse cognitive functioning, concentration issues, dropping out of school, repeating grades, and academic issues, including poorer reading performance. It is obvious that trauma exposure may cause aggressive and delinquent conduct as well as a decline in academic performance. Children who have been through traumatic experiences often have lower levels of academic accomplishment, including lowered IQ and reading skills, lower grade point average (GPA), and increased numbers of days missed from school.

According to research, reading proficiency suffers directly from exposure to violence. The researchers explained poor reading accomplishment by the fact that traumatized students are unable to leave their experiences outside of the classroom and bring them into their reading settings. Furthermore, when they don't feel protected, they find it difficult to focus on their schoolwork and instead become worried, afraid, and preoccupied with silencing the unpleasant memories. In addition, children who have experienced trauma have trouble with motivation, attention, focus, and interpersonal relationships—all of which are crucial for encouraging reading success.

Teachers must be aware of the impact trauma has on kids. I was hired at a school a few years ago for a program where I had to educate instructors on how to properly deal with various children in a classroom setting. I was surprised to see that many instructors did not show adequate consideration for students who had experienced trauma in their homes or had some other kind of trauma history. They were simply not trained to deal with kids with trauma history. A middle school teacher approached me after the program's completion to share her story.

"I didn't fully understand that kids' poor behaviors and learning impairments may be caused by underlying difficulties in their personal life until I attended your program and analyzed the effects of trauma on the mental health, cognition, learning, and behavior of children. In the past, I dealt with inappropriate behavior by imposing penalties right away, sometimes contacting the principal. Now that I am aware of the consequences of trauma on kids, I meet with students after behavioral issues occur, and we work together to figure out why they acted that way and also come up with a strategy for dealing with their emotions the next time the same situation occurs. Let's say, what can we do instead of shouting or fighting? Our strategy often incorporates the techniques you recommended in the program, including writing, painting, and other ways to vent their emotions and develop self-control. We also practice exercises like deep breathing and physical workouts. I'm glad I learned this because I believe this has made me a better teacher."

There is a lack of training for classroom instructors in the implementation of the intervention programs that are advised to help pupils in overcoming the consequences of trauma. If given the proper training, there are adjustments that instructors may make to their regular teaching methods and relationships with students to support them in succeeding despite their history of traumatic experiences.

Chapter 3: Tips to Deal with Trauma

Sophie, a 16 years old girl, came to see me at my clinic around two years ago. Despite the fact that Sophie was not there at the time of the tragedy, she discovered that she was reliving the last moments of her brother's life over and over again in her head. Her brother died in a car crash during a rainstorm.

"That story kept replaying in my thoughts, and I couldn't shake the feeling that I was stuck in a loop." She recalled that with each playback, she would agonize over whether or not her brother had any pain before passing away, and she would become progressively afraid that someone else might die. "The secure and predictable environment you formerly lived in is no longer available to you. When my brother passed away, I had the impression that my parents could no longer protect us. I believe my brother died suddenly, so I may also die suddenly."

Getting over a traumatic experience like Sophie's is not an easy task by any means. A few days or weeks may be enough time for some individuals to recover well and go on with their lives. While for others, the trauma can haunt them for a lifetime. Learning to cope with trauma early in a healthy manner is even more important for the fragile minds of teens.

It is important to learn the difference between healthy and unhealthy coping mechanisms. There are also situations in which behaviors that strictly speaking qualify as coping strategies do not result in favorable consequences. It's possible that some meals, like comfort foods, might help us get through tough times, but relying only on food as a coping method can have other, potentially detrimental effects on our health in the long run. In a similar vein, those who use drugs and alcohol as a form of self-medicating for the effects of traumatic experiences are, in a sense, coping, but they are setting themselves up for further difficulties in the future.

It is very necessary for trauma survivors to grant themselves permission to take more time for self-care and to seek out enjoyable activities that might provide them with a "break" from the intensity of their feelings. This entails ensuring that you are taking care of the fundamentals, such as obtaining enough amount of sleep, being hydrated, and keeping a healthy diet. But also seeking reasons to have optimism.

For instance, someone who, like Sophie, has been through a big loss could feel as if they have lost the ability to touch and be close to others. A session of acupuncture or massage can be just what's needed to satisfy this need. Activities that include movements, such as yoga or dancing, may be particularly beneficial. Trying out a new pastime or taking a class related to a hobby that you've always been interested in might be precisely helpful.

When individuals participate in good coping mechanisms, they often uncover a new sense of purpose or meaning in their lives. Attending memorial services for those who have passed away is another way to honor the memory of departed loved ones. Support groups have the potential to foster new levels of comprehension and even advocacy. Even while effective coping mechanisms might differ from person to person, the importance of having social support cannot be overstated. After experiencing a traumatic event, key risk factors for the development of a mental illness include social isolation, unemployment, and a lack of access to services that may provide help.

This chapter is going to help you discover many ways that you may use to cope with all the negative feelings related to trauma and the other post-traumatic effects.

3.1 Practice Self-Care

Self-care has been described as a comprehensive, multidimensional process of intentional participation in practices that support healthy functioning and improve well-being. Practicing self-care is profound for a trauma survivor.

The phrase self-care essentially refers to a deliberate action a person makes to improve their own mental, physical, and emotional wellness.

Self-care may come in a variety of ways. Making sure you receive adequate sleep each night or going outdoors for a little period of time to breathe some fresh air are two examples.

In order to develop resilience against the stressors in life that are unavoidable, self-care is essential. When you have put in the effort to take care of both your mind and your body, you will be in a better position to live the life you want to live.

Sadly, a lot of individuals see self-care as a luxury rather than a need. As a result, they are left feeling overburdened, worn out, and unable to deal with life's inevitable obstacles.

In order to make sure you are taking care of the body, mind, and spirit, it is crucial to evaluate how you are taking care of yourself in a number of different areas.

Finding methods to relax is just one component of practicing self-care. It is about taking care of yourself in all aspects of your life, including your mind, body, emotions, relationships, and soul. Finding a balance that enables you to take care of each of these areas is crucial for maintaining your health and well-being. There are times when you may need more self-care in a particular area in order to reestablish equilibrium or find relief from a stressor that is present in your life.

Physical Self-Care

If you want your body to function properly, you must take care of it. Remember that there is a close relationship between your mind and body. When you take care of your body, you'll notice improvements in the quality of your thoughts and feelings as well.

The way in which you refuel your body, the amount of sleep you receive, the amount of physical exercise you undertake, and the degree to which you tend to your own physical requirements are all aspects of how well you care for yourself physically. As part of proper physical self-care, it is important to keep all of your doctor's visits, take all of your medications as directed, and manage your health.

Asking yourself the following questions about your physical self-care will help you determine if there are any aspects of your routine that might need some improvement:

Are you getting enough rest?

How well is your body being fueled by your diet?
Are you making an effort to improve your health?
Are you exercising enough?

Social Self-Care

Participation in social activities is essential to good self-care. When life becomes hectic, though, it may be challenging to find the time to spend with friends, and it's simple to forget the ties you have with others.

Your well-being depends on having close relationships. Investing time and effort into developing meaningful connections with other people is the most effective strategy for establishing and sustaining meaningful friendships and romantic partnerships.

There is no predetermined amount of time that you need to spend cultivating your connections or spending time with your friends. Everyone's social demands are a little bit unique. The secret is to identify your social demands and allocate enough time in your calendar to achieve the ideal level of socialization.

To evaluate your social self-care, take the following questions into account:

How much face-to-face time do you spend with your friends on a regular basis?
How do you take care of your friendships and family ties?

Mental Self-Care

Your mental health is profoundly impacted, both directly and indirectly, by the thoughts that you think and the information that you let into your head.

Solving puzzles or learning about a topic that interests you are examples of mental self-care activities. Watching movies and reading books that inspire you may be something you find to be mentally energizing.

Practicing mental self-care also entails engaging in activities that contribute to maintaining mental wellness. For example, engaging in self-compassion and acceptance practices may assist you in sustaining a better internal dialogue.

When considering your mental self-care, keep the following questions in mind:

> Are you giving yourself enough time to engage in cognitively stimulating activities?
> Are you taking proactive measures to maintain your mental health?

Spiritual Self-Care

According to the findings of several studies, a lifestyle that makes room for religious or spiritual practices is typically one that promotes better health.

The cultivation of your spirit, however, does not necessarily need a religious practice always. It may consist of anything that contributes to the development of a deeper feeling of meaning, comprehension, or connection with the greater cosmos.

Self-care that focuses on your spiritual well-being is essential, and it doesn't matter whether you do it by praying, meditating, or attending a religious ceremony.

Think about your spiritual life and ponder these questions:

> What kind of queries do you pose to yourself about your life and the things you've experienced?
> Are you involved in spiritual activities that you find satisfying?

Emotional Self-Care

To cope with unpleasant emotions such as anxiety, fear, and grief, it's critical to have effective coping mechanisms. Activities that assist you in frequently acknowledging and safely expressing your emotions are examples of emotional self-care.

Emotional self-care should be a priority in everyone's lives, and it may take many forms. Some people find it helpful to discuss their feelings with a significant other or a close friend, while others find that engaging in leisure activities that enable them to work through their feelings is beneficial.

Consider the following questions as you evaluate the methods you use for your emotional self-care:

> Do you have a healthy and effective means of managing your emotions?

Do you make it a habit to engage in pursuits that may help you feel refreshed and revitalized?

3.2 Accept your Feelings and Emotions

Learning to accept and endure unpleasant feelings may be beneficial, especially if those feelings are painful or otherwise difficult to experience. Emotional acceptance emphasizes the significance of allowing these sentiments to exist and acknowledging that you are not harmed by them. This is in contrast to rejecting, denying, or otherwise attempting to suppress such feelings.

Acceptance frees you from the burden of having to choose between denying or suppressing your emotions or feeling powerless in the face of them. Instead, it enables you to concentrate on managing your emotions in constructive or healthy ways. If you do this, you will not only have a greater understanding of your feelings, but you will also have a better ability to manage them.

When you are confronted with an unpleasant emotion, such as grief, fear, or humiliation, your natural inclination is to want to push that sensation away as quickly as possible. You can convince yourself that you don't want to feel it if it seems like a "bad" emotion. Consequently, you can decide to engage in some activity in order to get rid of the sensation. This might mean attempting to ignore it or self-medicate with substances like drugs or alcohol in order to feel better.

Nobody wants to go through life constantly experiencing emotional agony, yet denying your feelings may sometimes make the situation much more difficult to deal with. Emotions have a variety of functions, one of which is to provide insightful information about the external environment. This indicates that it is not in anyone's best interest to suppress or bury their feelings in any manner.

Learning to embrace your emotional experiences is a better option than ignoring or suppressing your feelings. The term for this process is "emotional acceptance.

To practice acceptance is to train yourself to let your feelings just be what they are, without criticizing them or making an effort to alter them in any way.

It is crucial to differentiate between acceptance and rejection in all circumstances. Simply because you acknowledge and accept your feelings does not mean that you have to be miserable or dwell in your suffering forever. It also does not imply that you should strive to force yourself to experience emotional anguish or that you should try to cling to uncomfortable feelings.

Being aware of one's feelings and recognizing them for what they are in the present moment but also accepting them with the knowledge that they are not permanent is all that is required to practice acceptance.

Consider yourself a veteran of a lengthy war with your emotions as a metaphor for acceptance. Giving up your weapons and leaving the battle is the act of acceptance. You are not committing yourself to be beaten up by your emotions at any point in this process. Instead, you are only letting go of the battle that you have been going through.

Accepting one's feelings necessitates one's acceptance of the fact that such feelings are subject to change. When you are happy, you have to remind yourself that pleasure is a temporary state and that you should not expect to be happy all the time. This is true for every feeling, from happiness to sorrow to fear and worry. Feelings are ephemeral and may often be forgotten in a matter of seconds, hours, or days.

You may wonder why is it beneficial to acknowledge your feelings? It would be simpler to just get rid of your feelings, so what's the use of attempting to accept them? To answer this question, getting rid of emotions is not a simple task.

In point of fact, a lot of individuals have attempted to rid themselves of their feelings without much success. What they have discovered, and what is supported by research, is that it is extremely difficult, if not entirely impossible, to get rid of emotion in a simple manner.

Because there is a purpose to the existence of your feelings, you shouldn't make it your goal to eradicate all of them. Your feelings are a component of a more intricate system that assists you in making decisions on what you should avoid and what you should go toward. Emotions also have a role in the development of long-lasting connections with other individuals.

Neglecting one's feelings might result in making bad decisions. Therefore, acknowledging your emotions is beneficial as you may get useful knowledge by attending to what you are experiencing in the present moment.

3.3 Find Support and Process your Feelings

Every time you pick up the phone after a difficult day, accept assistance when you're overwhelmed, or simply seek online for advice on how to deal with a stressor, you're proving that you understand what science has repeatedly demonstrated: that various sorts of social support may truly help with stress! Getting social support and talking to a friend can be one way to process your feelings.

If other people are aware of your traumatic experience, there is a good probability that they will offer their assistance. Let your family and friends ease your burden by assisting with chores or lending a sympathetic ear. You will be able to return the favor at a later time when you are in a position to do so, and they are in need of anything.

However, it is important to keep in mind that not all forms of social support have the same effect on us. For example, having a lengthy conversation with a friend who is compassionate feels very different than having a conversation with someone who has a lot of advice to offer, and both of these forms of social support feel very different than the type of support that could be provided by a counselor or therapist. Is there a superior kind of social support than others? And how exactly do the various forms of social assistance influence our lives? It may be interesting for you to learn that there are four different kinds of social support, and each kind has something different to offer.

Emotional Support: This kind of assistance often entails providing some kind of physical comforts, such as by hugging the person or patting them on the back, in addition to actively listening and demonstrating empathy. To provide you with emotional support, a close friend or parent may offer you a bear hug, listen to your concerns, and let you know that they understand what you are going through.

Informational Support: Those who provide informational assistance do so either in the form of providing guidance or in the form of collecting and sharing information that might help others become aware of possible subsequent measures that may prove to be effective.

Esteem Support: Social displays of encouragement or confidence are examples of this form of support. Someone who is trying to boost your self-esteem could encourage you to see the positive qualities you have that you are overlooking or just let you know that they have faith in you. It is common practice for therapists and counselors to provide their clients with this kind of support in order to communicate to their clients that they have faith in them; as a result, clients often develop a stronger faith in themselves.

Tangible Support: One way to provide tangible support is to take on responsibilities for another person in order to help them manage a problem that they are going through. Another way to provide tangible support is to take an active stance in order to assist another person in managing a problem that they are going through. Someone who provides you with tangible support might bring you dinner when you're sick, assist you in coming up with potential solutions (instead of telling you what you should do, as is the case with informational support), or assist you in actively addressing the problem at hand in some other way.

All of these different kinds of social support may be effective, but not with everyone and not always in the same ways. People have different preferences for certain kinds, combinations, or sets of social support, and these choices might vary greatly.

According to research, having supportive and healthy relationships might help you feel less stressed and have better overall health. For the sake of your mental health, creating a group of dependable friends or even just one dependable connection might be crucial.

You may develop connections with others that are really helpful and lasting by using the following fundamental abilities.

Meet New People

It takes some effort but building a network of friends who are actually there for you may make a significant impact on how you manage stress and how you deal with life in general. The more individuals you have in your life, the greater the likelihood that you will have at least one connection with one of those people that is really helpful. Being able to often expand your network of friends is advantageous.

Make the Time

It might be challenging to carve out the time necessary to keep up with and extend your existing social group. You can always find time to hang out with your friends and family, even if your calendar is already jam-packed with other obligations and commitments. The most important thing is to acquire the skill of time management and organization.

Be Assertive

A common misconception about assertiveness is that it is the antithesis of passivity and involves "taking a stand for yourself" and "not letting others push you down." Although usually accurate, assertiveness also serves as a counterbalance to aggression. The key distinction is that when you express yourself, you don't have to sacrifice the needs of others in order to fulfill your own need.

Developing the ability to be assertive may be of great assistance in enhancing the quality of your relationships, helping to ensure that they are mutually supportive and long-lasting and that they open the channels of communication.

Listen

When you've had a long and challenging day, sometimes all it takes to change things around is to be able to vent to a reliable friend about how you're feeling. Having the experience of being heard and fully understood may have a significant impact on us.

Trust Your Intuition

Pay attention to how you feel when you are in the presence of specific individuals. If you feel comfortable with the other person or at ease in their presence, your gut instinct is probably letting you know that it's safe to interact with them.

On the other hand, if you leave an interaction with someone feeling worried, exhausted, or as if something is wrong with you, but you can't describe what it is, your intuition may be trying to warn you that you should avoid further interactions with that person.

You'll have better connections and a more robust social circle if you give consideration to the cues that your intuition gives you and take appropriate action on those indications.

3.4 Practice Grounding

The purpose of the coping approach known as grounding is to "ground" you in the current moment or to quickly link you with the here and now. When someone has gone through traumatic experiences or is diagnosed with post-traumatic stress disorder, grounding techniques are often utilized as a method of dealing with dissociation or flashbacks. These techniques may also be useful in the treatment of several other forms of anxiety disorders.

It is possible to classify grounding as a subset of mindfulness due to the emphasis placed on being fully present in the here and now. The use of grounding methods may also serve as a diversion, helping you to move away from troubling ideas, memories, or sensations.

The five senses—taste, sound, sight, smell, and touch—are often used in grounding practices because they enable you to rapidly reconnect with the here and now. For instance, grounding activities like singing, massaging moisturizer into your hands, and chewing on sour candies all provide sensations that are hard to ignore and hence are used as a diversion from your thoughts.

This enables you to connect with the here and now in a way that is both direct and immediate. Additionally, grounding lessens your chance of experiencing a dissociative or flashback episode.

The manner in which one grounds themselves is quite individual. What calms or soothes the anxiety or memories of one individual may do the opposite for another. It's possible that you won't know which grounding strategies work best for you until you give them a try and see what happens. Take note of the coping skills you've previously acquired to help you deal with flashbacks and anxiety, and consider if you can expand on them or utilize them as grounding strategies.

Grounding Techniques

Doing a single activity (or many activities) that will draw all of your attention to the current moment can help you connect with what is occurring in the here and now. It is important to remember to keep your eyes open while you are grounding yourself so that you can remain aware of everything that is occurring in your surroundings.

Try some of these tactics for grounding yourself in the present if you find that you are having flashbacks or entering a dissociative state.

Sight

Finish a puzzle such as a word search, crossword, sudoku, or another kind of puzzle.

Count how many different pieces of furniture there are in the room.

Take your mind off things by playing a game on your laptop, iPad, or smartphone.

Start one of your go-to movies or shows on television.

Take some time to read a magazine or a book.

Make a mental list of everything that is going on in your immediate environment, including all of the patterns and colors that you can see, the noises that you can hear, and the fragrances that you can smell. This may also be useful if you say it out loud.

Smell

Use some essential oils that bring back pleasant memories for you (such as those of freshly mowed grass, clean laundry, rain, or chocolate chip cookies, for example), and smell it.

Set a scented candle alight or melt some scented wax.

Take deep breaths of peppermint oil, which not only smells great but also has a calming effect on the body.

Sound

Make a call to a close friend or relative.

Play some natural noises like birds singing or the sound of waves smashing on the shore.

Read aloud whatever you're reading, whether it's your go-to book, a blog article, or a novel.

Talk out loud about the things that you are seeing and hearing, as well as the things that you are thinking and doing.

Play your favorite music loudly or turn up the radio.

Taste

Take a bite of something sour like a lemon.

Allow a chunk of chocolate to melt in your mouth as you pay attention to how it tastes and how it feels as you move it around on your tongue.

Try chewing some peppermint or cinnamon gum, sucking on a mint, or sucking on a minty candy.

Try putting some pepper on your tongue or some spicy salsa.

Touch

If you have a pet dog or a cat, pat it and cuddle with it.

Enjoy a warm or cold beverage.

Grab a piece of clothing, a comforter, or a towel, and either knead it in your hands or press it to your face. Focus your attention on the sensations you are experiencing while you're doing so.

Take an ice cube in your palm and let it melt while you hold it there.

Massage your temples.

Pop a piece of bubble wrap.

Run some water over your hands.

Notice the surface texture of a rug or a piece of furniture by softly rubbing your fingers over it.

Have either a warm or a cold shower.

Other

Dance to your favorite song.

Take a stroll or sprint around the block.

Write someone special in your life a note or send them a greeting card.

For a change of scenery, sit in a different room or location.

Do some leg, neck, and arm stretches.

Take ten long, slow, and deep breaths.

You might maintain a notebook and write about how you're feeling in it, or you could have a list of writing prompts on hand and use it to help you pick what to write about.

The fact that grounding may be done in a variety of settings is one of its many attractive features. You may employ grounding to bring your attention back to the here and now whenever you feel yourself about to have a flashback or experience dissociation, regardless of whether you are alone in your house or among other people.

Dedication is required while working on grounding, although the process becomes simpler with practice. If you find that these specific grounding strategies are not effective for you, you should look into other options. Some individuals, for instance, feel that wearing a rubber band on their wrist is helpful in bringing them back to the present moment when they get distracted. The end objective is to be able to live in the here and now and keep your attention on the present even when memories of the past begin to surface.

3.5 Maintain a Structure and Routine

Maintaining a routine in your life may be a beneficial method to safeguard your mental health while you are coping with traumatic events that have occurred in your life. When life seems to be out of your control, the routine might help you feel more focused and in charge of the situation. Keeping a regular schedule is quite important, especially for younger children and teens.

According to research, routines may be an effective tool for helping adolescents manage their anxiety and stress levels. When you are faced with the trials of life, keeping some sense of organization in your life may assist you in taking better care of both yourself and your health.

While some individuals look forward to the stability that comes with having a set routine each day, others cringe at the idea of being tied to a timetable. Keeping to a schedule and a routine, however, might make you feel less disorganized and more in charge, particularly during times of extreme stress.

It is true that having a routine may be beneficial at any time, especially if you are attempting to develop good habits; yet, these routines can be of utmost importance at times when elements of your life seem uncertain.

Feelings of unease may actually be made worse by a lack of structure and regularity, which can then direct your focus more intently to the root of the issues you are experiencing. People are likely to find themselves worrying about stressful situations more often if they do not have a framework to follow and are sitting about with less things to concentrate on. This may result in even greater feelings of stress and worry for the individuals involved.

Maintaining some kind of structure and regularity throughout the day is one strategy for breaking out of the loop that encourages you to keep thinking about the things that are causing you stress.

Research has repeatedly shown that routines may have a significant effect on the mental health of an individual. For instance, one research came to the conclusion that individuals might benefit from having routines in order to better manage their post-traumatic anxiety and stress.

Maintaining a consistent schedule may be of use to you in the following ways:

> It reduces your levels of stress.
> Develop healthy routines for each day
> Take greater care of your health;
> It makes you feel more focused and productive

Getting the daily tasks done in a scheduled manner will not only free up more time for you to engage in healthy habits, such as exercising, but it can also free up more time for you to enjoy pleasurable activities and hobbies.

The most important thing is to establish a schedule for yourself that provides your day with structure and a feeling that it can be anticipated. Maintaining a basic framework for the times at which you will get up, eat, study, engage in activities, and sleep will assist you in experiencing less stress and a greater sense of organization. Your schedule may shift somewhat from day to day, but this is to be expected, and keeping to this pattern can help you feel more organized and less stressed.

Organizing your day in this way also makes it more likely that you will complete the fundamental responsibilities that are obligatory, freeing up time for you to fit in additional activities that you either want to or are required to do.

Having a consistent schedule will make you feel more structured and productive, both of which will contribute to your sense of being more proactive and in control when confronted with a stressful scenario. Parents can help younger kids to build up a routine. However, older teens who are self-sufficient can come up with their own schedules.

There are a few things that, if included in your daily routine, may assist you in better managing the effects of stress. A few examples are as follows:

> Maintaining an active lifestyle and engaging in regular, everyday exercise
> Maintaining a healthy sleep schedule
> Maintaining a consistent eating routine that consists of nutritious meals
> Establishing goals that are attainable
> Trying to maintain an optimistic outlook
> Maintaining a schedule for study hours at home
> Preparing for problems but not dwelling on issues that are beyond your control
> Keeping in contact with loved ones, including family members and friends
> Putting aside time for things that you take pleasure in doing

Making a list of the activities that you often carry out throughout the course of a day might be a useful exercise.

Include anything from studying to preparing meals to doing tasks around the home. As soon as you have a concept of the fundamental responsibilities that need to be fulfilled, you can begin the process of developing a broad plan for what you would need to do each day in order to remain on schedule.

Since stress may make it difficult to concentrate, defining these everyday routines will assist you in better concentrating on what is most important.

Even while it is crucial to get the fundamentals done, you should make sure to find activities that you're excited to look forward to, such as calling a friend or enjoying your favorite TV show. When you are working on a job that you do not really love as much, it may be helpful to make these tiny incentives a regular part of your routine since these can help you stay positive and focused.

It is of equal importance to determine what strategy of scheduling tasks works the best for you. For some individuals, having a highly planned daily schedule that defines tasks in particular blocks of time may be the most productive way to organize their day, while for others, having a more general list of things they need to do throughout the day may be more effective.

How can you choose which strategy is most suited to your needs? Think about what you need to get done, as well as what is driving you to accomplish it. If it is something that has to be completed on a certain day, let's say an assignment, and is of great significance, then incorporating it into your daily routine and setting out time for it may be important to ensure that it gets done on time.

In other words, you should purposefully set up a certain amount of time in your calendar to deal with the activities that have the highest importance. The realization that you have allotted some time specifically for the completion of those important tasks will liberate you to concentrate on making the most of the other portions of your day.

3.6 Use Creative Methods for Expression

Art therapy refers to the practice of using creative exercises or activities in order to cure psychological conditions and improve mental health. Art therapy is a method that was developed on the premise that engaging in artistic expression helps promote physical and mental health recovery.

Since the beginning of time, people have turned to various forms of artistic expression for the purposes of communicating, expressing themselves, and finding healing. However, art therapy did not begin to develop into an established practice until the early 1940s.

As a result of the observation made by medical professionals that patients who were suffering from mental conditions often expressed themselves in some form of art like drawings and other artworks, a growing number of researchers started investigating the use of art as a therapeutic technique. Since that time, the practice of art therapy has grown to become an integral component of the wider therapeutic community and is included in certain evaluation and treatment strategies.

Art therapy seeks to leverage the artistic process as a means of assisting individuals in exploring new avenues of self-expression and, as a result of doing so, discovering novel approaches to gaining personal insight and developing innovative coping mechanisms.

Exploring one's feelings, being more self-aware, developing strategies for dealing with stress, improving one's sense of self-worth, and honing social skills may all be accomplished via the practice of creating or appreciating art.

The following are examples of methods that may be used in art therapy:

> Collage Making
> Painting
> A combination of doodling and scribbling
> Coloring
> Finger painting
> Photography
> Drawing
> Sculpting
> Creating things out of clay

During the course of the art-making process, teens may reflect on what they have created and how it makes them feel. They may search for themes and conflicts that could be influencing their ideas, emotions, and actions by looking at their work.

Art therapy is not the only form of creative expression that is used in the treatment of mental health conditions. The following are some examples of other creative forms of therapy:

Dance therapy: The use of movement in a psychotherapy setting to foster social, emotional, mental, and physical integration is referred to as dance/movement therapy, abbreviated as DMT. DMT has been shown to improve people's physical health in a number of ways, including enhancing strength and flexibility, lowering levels of muscular tension, and enhancing coordination. Additionally, it may bring substantial advantages to mental health, such as the decrease of stress and even the alleviation of symptoms associated with mental illnesses such as depression and anxiety.

DMT manifests itself differently for each individual based on their feeling of safety, their level of access to their bodies, and their individual level of comfort with an authentic expression of their bodies. The method might be mostly spoken or verbal or primarily nonverbal or motion-based. During a session of dance therapy, a therapist could do the following:

> Assist you in gaining an understanding of the link between the way you move and the feelings you feel.
> Encourage the monitoring of one's physiological feelings as well as one's breath.
> Assist you in navigating your way via spontaneous and self-expressive motions
> Provide particular therapeutic techniques, such as movement or vocal therapy to facilitate recovery.
> Assist you in working through the emotions that were triggered by the exercise.

Mirroring is a method that includes replicating the motions of another person and may be used in the field of dance therapy. People may find that doing so helps them feel more connected to other people and fosters sentiments of empathy as a result.

Expressive therapy: The purpose of supportive-expressive therapy is to assist people in gaining self-understanding, gaining mastery over their challenges, and practicing self-control with regard to their mental health issues. This therapy is mainly used for dealing with drug substance abuse, but it is also seen as helpful in treating trauma-related stress and anxiety. It is predicated on the idea that formative childhood experiences, such as those that shape a person's personality, have a role in the evolution of problematic drug use.

Drama therapy: The use of drama and/or theater methods, such as improvisation, role-playing, employing puppets, and acting out tales, is an integral part of drama therapy, which takes a novel approach to treat mental health conditions. It is an interactive and immersive kind of creative therapy that has the potential to assist you or someone you care about in gaining self-confidence and exploring new ways to solve problems.

The use of drama in conjunction with traditional psychotherapeutic techniques results in the provision of fresh avenues via which one may communicate their thoughts and feelings, hence facilitating improved behavioral and emotional health.

Writing therapy: Writing therapy is very effective with teens. Many therapists utilize it as a tool to assist teenagers in verbalizing their emotions via the use of written words. Writing therapy, which is also often referred to as journal therapy, involves using a variety of activities to build a conversation between teenagers and their therapists, with the goal of assisting teens in improving their mental, spiritual, and emotional well-being.

In the same way that there are therapists who specialize in art and music, there are also therapists who are trained exclusively in writing or journal therapy.

Writing for therapeutic purposes often comprises the following:

Poetry
Journaling
Narratives
Storytelling
Dialogue
Stories with humor

It is one way that may help reduce tension, figure out issues, work through difficult emotions, find connections between feelings and behavior, and a lot of other things.

It is very versatile and may be used for any issue or circumstance that a teenager is currently dealing with. According to the findings of recent studies, this kind of expressive therapy is an excellent method for enhancing one's mental and physical well-being.

Writing therapy is often used as a complementary modality to augment both group and individual therapy sessions. Teenagers may choose to write about traumatic events that are hard to talk about or difficulties that have been brought up during therapy.

Music therapy: Music therapy is a therapeutic method that makes use of the inherently mood-lifting aspects of music to help individuals improve their mental health and general well-being. This may be accomplished via the use of music in a variety of settings.

This is a goal-oriented intervention, which may entail the following:

> Making music
> Singing songs
> Writing songs
> Listening to music
> Dancing
> Discussing music

People who suffer from PTSD, anxiety, and depression may find that this kind of therapy is beneficial, and those who have issues with their physical health may find that it helps improve their quality of life. It is not necessary to have any prior training in music in order to benefit from music therapy; anybody may participate in this kind of therapy. This especially works well with teens.

3.7 Redirect your focus to what you can Control

When you are attempting to cope with the aftereffects of a traumatic event, you may experience feelings of powerlessness or helplessness, which may be both overwhelming and scary. One strategy for overcoming this challenge is to direct your attention to things that are within your power to influence.

When you take your attention away from the things that you have no control over or that you are unable to alter, you are better able to concentrate your efforts on the factors that are within your command and have the potential to make your circumstance more favorable. As you deal with the many sources of stress in your life, this might help you feel more in control and more robust.

Understanding the concept of locus of control is important here. The term "locus of control" refers to the degree to which individuals have the impression that they are in charge of the circumstances that have an impact on their life. Younger children and teenagers, in particular, need to be educated on the significance of developing an internal locus of control as early as possible in their lives.

Do you believe that you have influence over the result of a situation in your life while you are attempting to overcome a challenge? Or do you think that other people or events have more control over your life than you do?

Having what Psychologists call an "internal locus of control" means that you think you have some influence over the events that take place in your life. A person with what is termed as an external locus of control is one who believes that they do not have any influence over the events that take place and that others or circumstances outside of themselves are to blame.

Not only can your sense of control over situations in your life affect how you react to them, but it may also have an effect on how motivated you are to do something about them. If you feel that you have control over your own destiny, you are more likely to take action to alter your circumstances when it becomes necessary to do so. If, on the other hand, you feel that the result is beyond your control, you may be less inclined to make an effort to bring about change.

It is essential to keep in mind that the locus of control exists on a continuum. No one can claim to have a completely internal or external locus of control. In reality, most individuals are somewhere on a spectrum that may be found between the two extremes.

Individuals that have a dominating internal locus of control tend to exhibit the following qualities:

> They are more inclined to acknowledge and accept responsibility for the consequences of their conduct.
> They are often less affected by the thoughts and beliefs expressed by other individuals.
> They often do better in projects if they are permitted to work at their own speed.
> Have a healthy belief in one's own ability to succeed most of the time
> Usually, put forth a lot of effort to get the things that they desire.
> Have self-assurance in the face of difficult situations.
> Typically have a better level of physical health.
> Report feeling more content and self-sufficient.
> Often enjoy greater levels of success in their professional endeavors.
> Individuals that have a dominating external locus of control tend to exhibit the following qualities:

> They attribute their predicament to factors that are not within their control.

Usually attribute their triumphs to either luck or chance.

Do not think that they will be able to improve their circumstances by the actions that they do on their own.

Frequently experience feelings of hopelessness and helplessness in the face of challenging circumstances.

They are more likely to develop a sense of learned helplessness over time.

The terms "personal agency" and "self-determination" are often interchanged with the concept of "internal locus of control." While some studies have shown that males have a stronger internal locus of control than females, others have found the opposite — that females have a larger internal locus of control when compared to males. According to the findings of other studies, as individuals become older, they move toward having a locus of control that is more internal.

According to experts, those who have an internal locus of control often live happier lives. On the other hand, it is essential to keep in mind that an internal locus of control does not automatically equate to "good," nor does an external locus of control always equate to "bad."

Having a scenario that a person views as being beyond their control or one that constitutes a danger to their sense of self-worth are both examples of circumstances in which an external locus of control may be seen as a positive trait.

For instance, a teen who loses a sports game and has a strong internal locus of control may experience feelings of sadness or anxiety as a result of the loss. If he believes things like, "I'm not very good at sports, and I didn't strive as hard as I should have," he can let the defeat damage his self-image, which might cause him to feel anxious during future contests.

However, if he shifts his emphasis away from himself and onto the circumstances around him, such as saying to himself, "we were unfortunate to be paired with a stronger team," or "The weather wasn't in our favor!" he would likely experience a decrease in stress and a calm in his emotions.

3.8 Practice Deep Breathing

The practice of slow, deep breathing has been shown to be a very helpful strategy for reducing the negative effects of worry and stress. This kind of breathing is also known as diaphragmatic breathing, and it entails taking full, deep breaths from the diaphragm rather than taking short, shallow breaths from the chest.

People have a tendency to breathe more quickly and in a shallow manner when they are experiencing high levels of stress, which amplifies the body's reaction to worry. A feeling of relaxation may be induced in the body and brought about by breathing that is slower and deeper than normal.

You may be curious as to why "simply" breathing can have such an impact. The PNS or parasympathetic nervous system that is otherwise known as the "rest and digest" system of the body, is stimulated when one takes deep, slow breaths. It is responsible for restoring energy so that it may be utilized by the body for functions like urination and digestion.

Additionally, deep breathing stimulates the vagus nerve, which is said to be the "boss" of the parasympathetic nervous system (PNS). This system is responsible for regulating vital functions such as heart rhythm, digestion, and mood. In addition to this, it provides your brain and the rest of your organs with a greater amount of oxygen.

Before beginning an activity that requires deep breathing, you should check in with yourself for a moment and observe how you are feeling. Then, after completing the exercise, you should evaluate how you feel in comparison to how you felt before.

Practicing Deep Breathing Techniques

Following are two deep breathing techniques that you can practice in order to calm yourself down when experiencing stress or anxiety or some other post-traumatic effect.

Diaphragmatic Breathing

In the event that you are unfamiliar with the diaphragm, it is a tiny muscle that is located just underneath your lungs. It will constrict and move lower if you are breathing "properly," which will allow your lungs to expand and take in more fresh air. When you exhale, the reverse occurs, i.e., the muscle relaxes and moves higher up into your chest cavity.

> In order to practice diaphragmatic breathing:
> You should start by placing one hand over your chest and the other hand over your stomach.
> Take a deep breath in through your nostrils, and feel the air filling up your stomach as you do so. Maintain your position with one hand on your chest and the other on your stomach, and pay attention to how the

hand on your stomach moves while the hand on your chest should remain still.

As you exhale, pull your belly in toward your spine as if you were blowing out candles on a birthday cake. This will help you improve your core strength.

Sense how the hand that's been resting on your stomach returns to its starting position.

Start by going through this process three to five times and taking note of how you feel after each round.

4-7-8 Breathing

In this method of breathing, you will take a breath in for 4 seconds, then hold it for 7, and then release it for 8 seconds:

Similar to the starting position for the diaphragmatic breathing exercise, place one hand on your chest and the other hand on your stomach.

While you sense your diaphragm lowering, take one calm, deep inhale from your belly. As you take a breath in, count to 4 in your head.

When you reach the top, be sure to hold your breath and count to 7.

Exhale for 8 counts via your mouth, totally emptying your lungs.

Repeat between three and five times or as many times as necessary until you feel more relaxed.

You may think it's strange to set a timer or alarm to remind you to breathe, but doing so can help you make sure that you take advantage of the wonderful effects of deep breathing on a regular basis.

Try doing a few sets of deep breathing exercises every time your alarm goes off in the morning rather than turning over and reaching for your phone.

The most beneficial aspect of using breathing as a method to relax is that no one has to be aware that you are doing it; as a result, you may practice it whenever you like and anywhere you choose. For instance, teens may practice this while sitting in a bus or a car on their way to school.

There may be some locations or circumstances that you are aware are likely to cause you to feel stressed and anxious, such as waiting in line at the supermarket, being stuck in a traffic jam, or at a crowded restaurant. Before things get out of hand, breathe, and take a moment to give your brain some fresh oxygen. Practicing this can help you with calming down your nerves and feel better about your surroundings.

3.9 Tips for Parents to Deal with Traumatized Teen

To assist teenagers in recovering from traumatic experiences and adjusting to the changes that come with adolescence, developing connection is essential; nevertheless, developing a relationship is not always simple. A brain that has been traumatized interprets everything novel or out of the ordinary as a potential danger. As a result, regulations or protective interventions might seem like punishments, and those who strive to foster safety or trust are seen as being the ones who are behaving maliciously. Thus, developing a healthy connection with teens becomes a challenging task for parents.

This inherent lack of trust, when combined with the effort to link cause and effect and the emotional shifts that are characteristic of adolescence, may rapidly create a negative cycle that affects the whole family. Take the following example: Despite your repeated reminders, a kid goes out beyond curfew without fully understanding that doing so would result in them being grounded. Adolescent processes your punishment as a challenge to the sense of security that they have constructed for themselves, and as a result, they experience feelings of fear, anger, and confusion when they are grounded. They react with verbal aggression because they can't express these powerful feelings, and you react angrily because you're exhausted, frustrated, and overburdened.

You can see how fast this scenario may grow much worse and how it may turn into a vicious cycle that puts the parent and the adolescent against one another.

You may build a parenting approach that is more effective and compassionate by gaining a better knowledge of the influence that traumatic experiences and adolescence have on a teen's brain. This will allow you to stop the cycle before it even starts. Following are the three ways to achieve this:

1. Only step in when it's really essential: There are certain conflicts that are not worth engaging in. Regardless of whether the adolescent has been through a traumatic event in the past, has a disability, or has had other unfavorable events in their life, parenting a teenager may be tough. Teenagers strive for independence and want to learn more about themselves. As a parent, it is easy to get into the mentality that you need to correct every potentially troublesome behavior your child may exhibit.

Before you attempt to "fix" anything, take a moment to stop and think if this intervention is totally necessary: is this truly a chance for the two of you to learn something new or develop together? Will acting now prevent a worse issue later? Do you possess the patience and skills necessary to manage this circumstance in a way that is both successful and efficient?

Keep in mind that you are the one who teaches your kid the skills necessary for them to be kind, creative, respectful, and polite. It's sometimes necessary to have faith in these skills that you have taught to your kid.

On the contrary, you shouldn't automatically assume that a shy, well-behaved adolescent doesn't need any kind of assistance or support. Compliance does not always signal progress or healing, and your kid may be hurting more than you think.

2. Focus on strengthening your connection: You need to be resourceful when you make the decision that it is time to intervene. Teens who have been through traumatic experiences may not always be fearful of or able to absorb punitive consequences because they are unable to link the cause with the effect, and they have already endured considerable loss in their lives. To put it another way, the "threat" of removing a kid's access to electronic devices, time spent with friends, and other privileges will not properly address a teen's conduct, and it may even serve to re-traumatize the youngster. Teenagers may really be mainly concerned with maintaining their self-esteem; thus, penalties, confrontations, and threats of dismissal will often simply make matters worse.

Realize that successful intervention for adolescents is not the intervention that forcefully eliminates behaviors; rather, it is an intervention that establishes a deeper connection and allows teenagers to grasp the depth of your love and care for them while giving them the opportunity they need to learn from their errors and blunders.

Therefore, structure your consequences around fostering relationships. Instead of isolating children from their peers and family members via practices such as "time out" and "grounding," consider having them serve their penalties by spending time with their families. While it may not be the best way for many teenagers to spend their weekend going on hikes or boat rides, dinner dates, or other adventures with grandparents, parents, or siblings but it can provide an effective penalty for bad conduct while still building relationships and conveying that regardless of what they do, you remain in their life for good.

A lot of parents think that positive behaviors should be rewarded with opportunities to participate in activities like attending a sporting event or having friends around. Rather, they are great tools to develop connections with others, assist healing, and model appropriate conduct! Let your children participate in extracurricular activities. Create a welcoming environment in your house so that your friends will want to come over. Find ways for adolescents, such as via volunteer work or taking care of a pet or other animal, to help them understand the needs of others. Find methods for your adolescent to laugh, sing, play, dance, and move about; all of these activities serve to mend trauma at its most basic level and help kids build a feeling of belonging, trust, and self-worth. Having fun as a family is one of the most important things you can do as a parent for your child.

When a kid becomes older, society views them as more accountable for their actions, which means that their parents and other caregivers lose greater control over the repercussions that a teen could face from the outside world. For instance, a teen might be expelled from the school if he scores a failing grade in any of his classes. In such a situation, keep in mind that it is your responsibility to convey to your kid that you love him completely and unconditionally and you're there to help him.

3. Work together as a team: Your relationship is a collaboration between you and your kid. So your kid deserves to be treated as an active participant in their own recovery journey. Include your kid in the decision-making process about consequences, treatment alternatives, activities, and other related matters by giving them a choice. You may want to consider giving them a choice between two or more alternatives that you have already pre-approved.

Offer them the opportunity to engage in this partnership by providing them with the language and space they need. As puberty and traumatic events may lead the "thinking" region of the brain to become disconnected from the "feeling" region of the brain, it can be challenging for adolescents to find words that adequately express their feelings or experiences. As a consequence of this, actions become the main mechanism through which emotions are communicated, and what would seem to be rebellious conduct is really simply a method of processing a problem. Take a step back and allow the youngster to explain, in their own words, what they believe happened rather than asking why something happened. Ask them what it is that they need, how they are feeling at present, and what other choices they have open to them for the next time something similar takes place. You should go at their speed, stopping and taking a step back if you see that they are becoming overwhelmed or uncomfortable with the situation. It is best to avoid having these discussions in the heat of the moment or in hostile circumstances, when a youngster may feel pressured to fill the silence or maintain eye contact, which might leave them feeling overwhelmed. Consider the possibility of initiating a conversation during an activity that involves movement, such as going for a stroll around the neighborhood, playing a game of soccer, or driving to dinner. This will allow you both to process your immediate feelings without feeling rushed or pressured to respond.

Finally, keep in mind that each successful collaboration demands a reciprocal exchange of favors. Give your adolescent the opportunity to learn and improve their caring and listening skills by expressing your own feelings to them as well. It may seem weird to cry in front of your kid or to communicate how you are feeling, but establishing this honesty enables them to know how much you care about them. Not only is this a key phase in the process of forming relationships, but it is also a significant method of demonstrating trust.

Chapter 4: Therapeutic Approaches and Interventions for Trauma Recovery

Throughout history, those who have survived traumatic experiences have not had a simple path to recovery. After World War II, mental health professionals, doctors, and the general public were at a loss to explain why veterans who had been in combat had such a hard time readjusting to life after the war. Soldiers often reported suffering from nightmares and flashbacks as a result of their experiences in war, which caused them to feel emotionally disconnected from other people.

This condition was first described to the general public as "shell shock." There was, in general, very little comprehension or awareness about human responses to potentially life-threatening circumstances. Following the end of the Vietnam War, there was a resurgence in the desire to assist those who had made it through horrific experiences of war. Since then, specialists in the field of mental health have started to get a better understanding of the typical ways in which individuals deal with a variety of traumatic situations, such as an incidence involving violence, sexual assault, or natural disasters. There has been a significant amount of work done to assist individuals of all ages, especially younger children and teenagers, in recovering from trauma and living a life that is not constrained by the symptoms of trauma or post-traumatic stress disorder (PTSD).

Cognitive behavioral therapy (CBT), Acceptance and Commitment Therapy (ACT), and Dialectical Behavior Therapy (DBT) are the three kinds of therapeutic approaches that may assist with the symptoms of PTSD and Anxiety. In this chapter, I will briefly describe these therapies. CBT is a treatment for PTSD that is supported by evidence. The acceptance and commitment therapy (ACT) has been shown to be effective in treating anxiety, while the dialectical behavior therapy (DBT) has been shown to be effective in assisting individuals in dealing with challenges in controlling their mood and building meaningful connections.

Each of these treatments includes fundamental beliefs about how individuals evolve, as well as certain core methods. In the later section of this chapter, I'll include some strategies from these approaches that teens may easily put into practice. Understanding the fundamentals can help you identify which strategies work best for you and help you choose which tactics to attempt. Getting educated is a crucial step in taking back some of your life's control and recovering from your trauma.

4.1 Cognitive Behavioral Therapy

People's feelings, thoughts, and emotions are the primary focal points of cognitive-behavioral therapy. It is predicated on a few essential assumptions, which are as follows:

• There is a connection between emotions, thoughts, feelings, and one's bodily responses. If we make a change in one, it will allow us to make adjustments in the others.
• Change occurs in little increments; it does not occur all at once.
• Changing behavior involves practice and is more complicated than just making a decision to do something.
• Labeling our actions as "good" or "bad" doesn't help us go forward in any way. It is more beneficial to think about

how our conduct fits in with our overall objectives. Or in other words, we should look at our behavior in terms of "healthy or unhealthy" and "helpful or not helpful."

Let's take a look at what cognitive-behavioral therapy (CBT) truly entails when it's put into practice. This particular example focuses on the feelings of sorrow and depression, which are common reactions to traumatic experiences and PTSD. It's possible that a friend who means well would tell you, "You need to pull yourself out of this depression; it's not healthy for you to be this depressed all the time." The reality is that if you could make yourself feel better by waving a magic wand, you probably would. Although it might be challenging to alter your feelings, you can frequently improve your emotional state by making adjustments to your thinking and your behavior.

In the event that you are suffering from depression, there is a possibility that your feelings are interfering with your ability to carry out everyday tasks. Perhaps one of your goals is to wake up early, prepare a healthy breakfast for yourself, and then head off to school. Perhaps signing up for a school sports team or a yoga class after school is one of your long-term objectives. When you're depressed, it might all seem a little overwhelming. The question is, where do you begin? Your greater long-term objectives may become more manageable if you use a cognitive behavioral therapy (CBT) approach.

The easiest way to make a change in your habit would be to commit to getting out of bed, brushing your teeth, and changing your clothes before 7:00 a.m. on three separate mornings this week. After altering your behavior in this little way for a period of two weeks, you'll see that, by the time 8:00 in the morning rolls around, you feel a little less gloomy and a little more attentive. You start to think to yourself, "In a couple of months, I'll be able to try out for the sports team." Using this scenario as an example, we can see how making very few adjustments to one's conduct may begin to disrupt the vicious cycle that links unfavorable ideas, poor actions, and emotions.

4.2 Dialectical Behavior Therapy

An intervention that shows a lot of promise for the treatment of trauma is dialectical behavior therapy (DBT). It has been shown to be particularly successful in helping individuals who have trouble controlling their emotions and building strong connections, as well as helping those who have thoughts of harming themselves. Dialectical behavior therapy places a strong emphasis on emotions and, more specifically, how we learn to manage challenging feelings. DBT might be extremely helpful to you if you have ever discovered that you are overpowered by challenging emotions and if those emotions cause problems in your interactions with other people. This approach to treatment involves a number of components, such as the development of abilities in mindfulness and interpersonal effectiveness, as well as management and tolerance of negative emotions. The following presumptions serve as the foundation for it:

•   If your emotional responses are ignored by your caregivers when you are a child, you may have trouble recognizing, naming, and managing your feelings as an adult. This may make it difficult for you to form relationships.

• Your connections with other people will suffer if you have trouble controlling your emotions and expressing them appropriately.

• When we dwell on the negative things that have occurred in the past as well as those that could take place in the future, our level of anxiety often rises.

• Mindfulness skills, which are a collection of strategies that enable you to come back to the here and now, may assist you in managing painful emotions and thoughts.

• There are times when it is beneficial to make an effort to modify unfavorable emotions, and there are other times when it is beneficial to accept those challenging emotions. You may build abilities that will assist you in selecting which option to adopt in a variety of different scenarios.

Let's look at an example of how mindfulness, one component of DBT, might assist you in managing trauma-related symptoms. Jessica was a victim of sexual abuse when she was a kid and managed to survive it. When she was ten years old, a neighbor sexually assaulted her three different times over the course of a year. Jessica attempted to tell her mom about the assault, but her mother did not believe her and said that Jessica "must have misinterpreted what occurred." She shared with Jessica that their next-door neighbor was a well-respected community member and that he cherished time spent with young children. Jessica was twelve years old when the abusive neighbor moved away, but she feels that the assault and her mom's response to it had a negative impact on her emotions of self-worth even after the neighbor had gone away.

At the age of nineteen, Jessica tied the knot with a guy who later turned out to be highly violent to both her and their children physically.

Jessica filed for divorce from her spouse when she was twenty-seven years old. She does not get any financial assistance from her ex-husband for the care of her children, who are now five and six years old. At the legal office where Jessica has worked for many years, she was recently given the opportunity to advance to the position of executive assistant. The job is both interesting and demanding in terms of the obligations it entails. Jessica does, however, sometimes have a very difficult time focusing. She claims that her thinking is "cloudy and dazed," and she is concerned that her inability to concentrate may result in her being dismissed from her job. Jessica has made the decision to practice various forms of mindfulness in order to assist her in regaining her attention and focus while she is working.

She engages in a variety of disciplines, but the ones that seem to be of the greatest use to her are the ones that focus on her sense of touch. Jessica plants both of her feet firmly on the floor whenever she notices that she is beginning to feel disoriented as a result of thinking about the assault. She pays close attention to the laptop's and desk's hard surfaces. She feels chilly and smooth as she runs her fingertips over a paperweight she has on her desk. After focusing on these feelings for about a minute, Jessica is finally able to bring herself back to the present and tell herself that she is no more a little girl of ten years old and that she is no longer living with her violent ex-husband. In this way, she is able to root herself in the here and now, which is a time of safety, and ultimately work her way towards calmness.

4.3 Acceptance and Commitment Therapy

Acceptance and commitment therapy, commonly known as ACT, is a method of psychotherapy that assists individuals in observing their thoughts and feelings in a non-judgmental manner. It stresses the need to determine your values and act on them, regardless of how you are feeling on the inside. The goal of ACT (acceptance and commitment therapy) is not to alter one's ideas or emotions; rather, the treatment places emphasis on the ways in which altering one's conduct may lead to a more fulfilling and satisfying existence. Your capacity to perceive events from a variety of perspectives and be resilient in the face of adversity may be improved by participation in this kind of psychotherapy, which helps you build psychological flexibility. The following are some of the presumptions that constitute acceptance and commitment therapy:

• We have the ability to learn to watch our own thoughts, feelings, and painful memories without being excessively immersed in the content of these experiences.
• When we accept our thoughts and emotions, we minimize the amount of emotional pain we experience because we stop making the fruitless effort to alter our own internal conditions.
• The skill of mindfulness may be of use to you while you work on developing acceptance.
• Your actual or true self is an aspect of you that is distinct from your thoughts or actions. This is something that

some individuals may refer to as their "soul" or their "essence."

• It is essential to first determine what you actually value and then to make efforts to conduct yourself in a manner that is congruent with those values.

The individual receiving ACT may get assistance with non-indulgence in experiential avoidance as one component of the therapy. Teenagers avoid not just what's going on inside but also the exterior events, such as social events, school assessments, and family activities that have the potential to serve as a "trigger" or signal for unwelcomed happenings on the inside. Avoiding situations that don't feel good is a normal human response, and it's effective. When we avoid unpleasant sensations and ideas, we experience a temporary reduction in those feelings and thoughts, which in turn reinforces our tendency to avoid them. This is known as experiential avoidance. Experiential avoidance may, however, be destructive when employed excessively and in ways that restrict our lives and undermine our feeling of purpose.

Consider the case of Sarah, a young girl of 15 years of age. Since Sarah was not very good at arithmetic, her math instructor used to make fun of her in front of the other students in the classroom when she was 13 years old. This caused Sarah a lot of embarrassment. Sarah now suffers from a great deal of anxiety as a direct result of going through traumatic experiences over the course of a year. She hardly passed the Math exam and feels that she is dumb. Her academic performance and social life have both suffered as a result of the stress. The mere prospect of upcoming examinations and tests is enough to send her into an anxious state. She is intent on avoiding the feelings of worry and dread, as well as the physical symptoms that are associated with her anxiousness.

Her anxiety levels rise whenever she considers upcoming academic tests, assignments, and social events, and she is always searching for new methods to alleviate her symptoms. Sarah's mind seamlessly connects the dots between tests, assignments, and social activities. She does all in her power to avoid participating in activities in the classroom that involve a collaborative effort, such as working on group projects. Simply considering any one of these things may lead to avoidance behavior and, as a consequence, a decrease in anxiety. But this behavior only makes her feel better for a short time. Her anxiety and fear come back when she still has tests to take, and she is always afraid that the school will call her about the projects she missed. So in the long term, Sarah's experiential avoidance does not help her.

4.4 Psychological Techniques and Exercises

People who have experienced traumatic events may now be helped in more ways than ever before. Techniques within CBT, DBT, and ACT have been shown useful for the treatment of PTSD and other symptoms related to traumatic experiences. You have read about some of these techniques, like deep breathing, in the previous chapter. This section is going to list a few more techniques to practice.

• **Getting Active**

Purpose: Creating an attainable objective and committing to a regular exercise regimen, such as stretching or yoga, is the purpose of this exercise.

Instructions: I'll start with an example to show you how the technique works. After that, establish your objective and log your activity session.

For example, I aim to spend 10 minutes stretching and doing ten pushups four times this week.

Exercise: I aim to _____ (add your activity here) for _____ (enter your time period here)

• **Progressive Muscle Relaxation**

Purpose: The goal of this exercise is to help you distinguish between relaxation and tension in your body so that you can stop the buildup of muscular tension before it becomes severe.

Instructions: Ensure that you are in a relaxed posture and begin by sitting in a chair. In accordance with the instructions that follow, tense and release each of the muscle groups individually. It is important to pay close attention to the differences in the emotions of relaxation and tension in each group of muscles. Wait 10 seconds in each tensed posture before moving on to the next. Hold for 10 seconds, then gently release your grip. Take note of the changes that occur in your muscles between the stressed and relaxed states. Check your anxiety levels before each practice session, and do so again afterward. Use a scale that goes from 0 to 10, where 0 represents the complete absence of anxiety and 10 represents extreme levels of anxiety.

1. Contract your toes by bringing them in toward the soles of your feet and curling them inward. You may release them by allowing them to return to their regular position.

2. Contract your ankles by pointing your toes toward the roof of the room while keeping your heels planted firmly on the floor. Release them by allowing them to fall back down to the ground.

3. Contract your calf muscles and your quadriceps (the muscles on the front of your thighs) by squeezing them. Release them fully.

4. Contract your gluteus muscles (the group of muscles that make up your buttocks) as tightly as possible. Release.

5. Contract the muscles in your abdominal region by drawing your stomach in as far as you possibly can. Bring your belly button back to its original position.

6. Contract the muscles in your back while drawing a long, deep breath into your chest. Release as you let your breath out.

7. Pull your shoulder blades closer together and squeeze them together to tighten your upper back and shoulders. Release.

8. Contract your shoulders and neck by bringing your upper back and shoulders closer to your ears. Relax and allow your shoulders to fall back into a comfortable posture as you let go.

9. Clench both of your fists tightly. Release the tension in your fingers by allowing them to return to their normal, slightly curved position.

10. Extend your arms and "make a muscle" in your biceps and tighten it. You may release simply by letting go of your arms.

11. Contract the muscles in your forehead by drawing your brows together and raising them as high as they will go. Release.

12. Squeeze your face together as tightly as you can while keeping your eyes closed, and then feel the muscles that surround your eyes. Let go, and start to open your eyes.

13. Make a "kissing" look by puckering your lips in an exaggerated manner. Relax your lips and jaw as you release the tension in the muscles that surround them.

• **Engaging the Senses**

Purpose: To develop a particular goal incorporating sensory awareness in your everyday life by utilizing several sorts of imagery (sight, smell, sound, touch, and taste).

Instructions: The five exercises are listed below. Try to picture each scenario as you read each one carefully.

Sight Exercise: Imagine yourself on a brown sand beach for this sight exercise. You can see the sand turning deeper and darker as you approach the coast because it is being saturated with ocean water. The water is sparkling and transparent. There is water as far as the eyes can see when you gaze toward the horizon. You can see the vivid orange sunshine as you gaze out over the bright blue sea and the beautiful blue sky.

Sound Exercise: You can hear the wind softly rustling the leaves as you go through the forest. You come to a halt when you hear a distant sound of a tiny squirrel scurrying over dry, crunchy leaves. Then there is total silence. The sound of your watch ticking may be heard in the background, along with the soft sound of your breath as it enters and leaves your body.

Touch Exercise: After waking up, place your hands in a bowl of cold water. As they are submerged in water, your hands seem airy and light. Your face is splashed with the chilly water. You may feel the cool water falling down your cheeks and eyelashes. You have the sensation of having a plush and warm towel pressed against your face. You feel revitalized when your fan's cold air blows on your cheeks.

Taste Exercise: You are presented with a large dish of your own homemade freshly baked cookies. You can taste the luscious chocolate chips and the mouthwatering butter flavor when you bite into a cookie. The cookie is tender and melts on your tongue since it just came out of the oven. Each mouthful of the cookie is enjoyable.

Smell Exercise: You are strolling through a lovely rose garden. The aroma of the flowery sweetness is present. You can see some lovely lilacs nearby. You can distinguish between the strong rose scent and the subtle lilac aroma when you take a breath.

• **Observing Painful Thoughts**

Purpose: The goal is to develop the ability to objectively notice your thoughts.

Instructions:

1. Pick a peaceful location free from distractions. Choose a setting in which you have a sense of being fairly secure.

2. Take a seat in a comfortable chair. Depending on how it feels, you may either have your eyes completely closed or opened. Set a five-minute timer.

Keep track of the ideas that come and go through your head. You don't have to consider if the ideas are true or untrue or what they imply. Just watch them. Pick an effective metaphor for the ideas and their passage, such as:

> **a.** You find yourself floating in the air on a cloud. It is supple and cozy. Consider a scenario in which all of your thoughts are on other clouds in the sky. You may observe them as they pass by. Just watch them. Follow their movements. There is no need for you to concern yourself with the specifics of the substance of any idea since you are protected on your cloud.

> **b.** Your chair is at the beach, and you're relaxing there. Think of your thoughts as waves. You observe them as they come and go along the shore. You can feel the sand under your feet. Some waves are calm, pausing as they approach the coast. Then they move away. Some waves reach the beach with great strength and vigor. These waves rapidly go away. As you sit comfortably on the shoreline, you can just watch the different waves.

- **Making a Metaphor for Change**

Purpose: The goal is to develop your own change metaphor, which will help you see your trauma-related thoughts from a new angle and will motivate you to deal with challenging circumstances and feelings. Both metaphors that highlight altering and controlling your circumstances, as well as metaphors that highlight your willingness to face painful emotions, are possible. Try out different metaphors to see which one suits you best.

Instructions: Read the illustration below. Then, develop your own metaphor for confronting the specific trauma-related circumstances, ideas, and emotions you steer away from. If you are having problems starting, consider an activity, item, or location that you like or find inspirational and utilize it to guide the metaphor's construction.

Example: My metaphor for transformation or change is a garden. I believe I should see my life as a garden. I would have adored a garden bursting with vegetables and blooms. But I am aware that the majority of my yard is too shaded and dry to grow lettuce. I'm going to be content with my garden, where I can see that the grass is healthy and green and that there are a few yellow dandelion plants on the boundaries.

• **Writing about Traumatic Experiences**
Purpose: The goal is to cease avoiding trauma-related thoughts and memories and to develop healthy coping mechanisms for uncomfortable flashbacks.

Instructions: Write down your traumatic experience in as much detail as you can. Rate your degree of distress before and after the writing on a scale from 0 to 10, where 0 represents no distress, and 10 represents extreme distress. Do this three times each week. Prior to and after each session, rate your degree of distress. Compare your evaluations two weeks later. You'll notice that your levels of distress are decreasing.

- **Mindfulness and Grounding Skills**

Purpose: The goal is to employ mindfulness and grounding techniques to return to the present moment both during and after distressing flashbacks and recollections.

Instructions: Try one of the methods below the next time you have a distressing flashback or recollection. What do you now hear, taste, feel, see, and smell? Pay as much attention to the details as you can. By utilizing nearby items or noises, you may develop your own methods to assist you in maintaining present-moment awareness.

Techniques to Try:

1. Take a look outside the window and note what you see.

2. Take a look around and attempt to describe the hues of the walls, carpet, and other elements in your immediate surroundings.

3. Pay attention to the wall clocks' ticking.

4. Be aware of your breathing.

5. Pay attention to the noises around you and attempt to explain them.

6. Feel the ground under your feet. Pay close attention to the areas of your feet that are touching the ground.

7. Feel your body seated in the chair, with your legs contacting the seat and your back against the back of the chair.

8. Touch anything in your pocket or bag and carefully explain how it feels.

9. Sense the touch of the air on your arm. Take note of the feeling and the temperature.

10. Touch your hair and face with your fingertips and notice how it feels.

11. Smell the fragrance of a relaxing perfume or lotion that you always carry.

12. Take a deep breath and smell the scents of the air around you. Take note of the temperature.

13. Smell the aroma of an apple, lemon, or orange. Pay attention carefully and describe the smell.

14. Take a sip of a cold beverage and notice how it feels in your mouth.

15. Chew on some gum or a mint and notice how it tastes and feels on your tongue.

Conclusion

A range of responses is possible for an individual who is confronted with traumatic experiences. A person may experience denial, shock, or a deep state of sadness as a result of the circumstances. In addition to the immediate or short-term response, trauma may also give rise to a variety of long-term reactions, such as emotional dysregulation, having nightmares, lack of impulse control, flashbacks, and the effects on relationships. These responses can last for much longer than the immediate or short-term reaction. These long-term effects are able to manifest themselves even years after the first stressful incident that triggered them. Those who have gone through traumatic situations may also exhibit bodily symptoms, such as exhaustion, headaches, and nausea, in addition to the psychological symptoms that they have experienced. Some people might experience much greater effects than others. When a traumatic incident has a significant impact on a person, they may find it difficult to go on with the rest of their lives because they are emotionally bound by the trauma. Post-traumatic stress disorder (PTSD) is a psychological condition that may occur when trauma manifests itself over an extended period of time.

Younger children and adolescents who have been through traumatic situations are more likely to have issues with their brain development, particularly with the development of the skills related to executive functioning. Teenagers who have been exposed to traumatic situations may have more difficulty learning certain abilities, such as the ability to manage their time effectively and organize their routines, the ability to control their impulses, to make judgments, and then act in line with those judgments. Traumatized teens may also have trouble keeping track of the information and being able to retrieve it when needed as well as displaying appropriate behavioral or emotional responses.

Given the many challenges, teens and their caregivers should work together in order to deal with all the after-effects of trauma. This book has provided you with all the important information that you may need to learn about trauma. I have also gathered some basic and easy techniques that a teen may utilize to deal with symptoms related to trauma. It is important to take small steps in order to cope with trauma effectively. Use the strategies given in this book and say goodbye to your inner fears.

Printed in Great Britain
by Amazon

24252288R00066